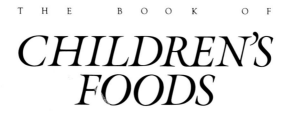

T H E   B O O K   O F

CHILDREN'S FOODS

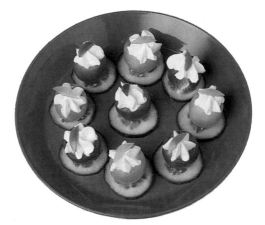

THE BOOK OF

CHILDREN'S FOODS

LORNA RHODES

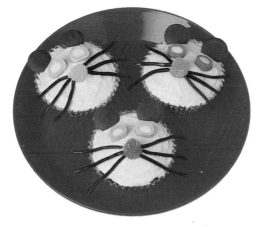

Photographed by
SUE JORGENSEN

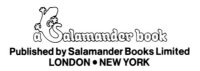
a Salamander book
Published by Salamander Books Limited
LONDON • NEW YORK

Published 1992 by Salamander Books Limited
129-137 York Way, London N7 9LG, United Kingdom

© Salamander Books Ltd 1992

ISBN 0 86101 650 5

Distributed by Hodder & Stoughton Services, PO Box 6,
Mill Road, Dunton Green, Sevenoaks, Kent TN13 2XX

Managing Editor: Felicity Jackson
Art Director: Roger Daniels
Editor: Louise Steele
Photographer: Sue Jorgensen
Home Economist: Lorna Rhodes
Typeset by: BMD Graphics, Hemel Hempstead
Colour separation by: Scantrans Pte. Ltd, Singapore
Printed in Belgium by Proost International Book Production

ACKNOWLEDGEMENTS

The Publishers would like to thank the following for their
help and advice:
Josie Firmin of Cosmo Place Studio, 11 Cosmo Place, London WC1, who kindly
provided plates.
Cannon Industries Ltd., Gough Road, Coseley, Bilston,
West Midlands WV14 8XR, for loan of the hob.
Kerry's Kitchen Shop, 119 King Street, London W6, and 417 Upper
Richmond Road West, London SW14, for loan of kitchen equipment.
Braun (UK) Ltd. for loan of the food processor and blender.

Companion volumes of interest:

The Book of SOUPS
The Book of COCKTAILS
The Book of CHOCOLATES & PETITS FOURS
The Book of HORS D'OEUVRES
The Book of GARNISHES
The Book of BREAKFASTS & BRUNCHES
The Book of PRESERVES
The Book of SAUCES
The Book of DESSERTS
The Book of ICE CREAMS & SORBETS
The Book of GIFTS FROM THE PANTRY
The Book of PASTA
The Book of HOT & SPICY NIBBLES-DIPS-DISHES
The Book of CRÊPES & OMELETTES
The Book of FONDUES
The Book of CHRISTMAS FOODS
The Book of BISCUITS
The Book of CHEESECAKES
The Book of CURRIES & INDIAN FOODS
The Book of PIZZAS & ITALIAN BREADS
The Book of SANDWICHES
The Book of SALADS
The Book of GRILLING & BARBECUES
The Book of DRESSINGS & MARINADES
The Book of CHINESE COOKING
The Book of CAKE DECORATING
The Book of MEXICAN FOODS
The Book of ANTIPASTI
The Book of THAI COOKING
The Book of AFTERNOON TEA

Notes:
All spoon measurements are equal.
1 teaspoon = 5 ml spoon
1 tablespoon = 15 ml spoon.

CONTENTS

INTRODUCTION

Cooking for children can be fun as they love brightly-coloured food and are often happy with the most simple creations. However, in our ever-changing world, children are now exposed to a wider variety of food than ever before – indeed many are fortunate enough to have travelled with their parents and sampled foreign dishes. Gone are the days when school children were given nursery food as a matter of course; now they often also like many of the sophisticated dishes their parents enjoy.

As parents we are responsible for giving children the best start possible in life, and an important contribution to this aim is making available wholesome, fresh foods. A balanced diet is important for everyone, but starting children off with good eating patterns and encouraging them to eat plenty of fruit and vegetables, and less fatty foods, is the best investment we can make for their future health.

This book has a stunning selection of recipes for children of all ages, with enticing dishes for the under fives, plus grown-up ideas for old children. For those children who enjoy cooking, with parental approval, the recipes are easy to follow, especially with the help of the step-by-step photographs. Older children will also love helping prepare the fun ideas for younger brothers and sisters, especially when it's for a birthday party or a special tea-time treat. Most of the recipes have been chosen with everyday eating in mind, but there are also delicious treats to make for those special celebrations.

It often seems an easy option to choose commercially prepared food, such as fish fingers and beefburgers, for the family; but what could be nicer and more wholesome than home-made fish cakes or a freshly-made pasta dish?

The recipes included help offer lots of interesting ideas for healthy meals, using the foods children enjoy.

With over 100 delicious recipes, all illustrated in full colour and with step-by-step instructions this book will appeal to people of all ages who love cooking and eating delicious food.

FOOD FOR CHILDREN

Food for children should be fun, with family meals a pleasant and relaxed occasion, but it is equally important that they learn to enjoy the taste of fresh and wholesome foods at an early age. This can easily be achieved by presenting food in novel and unusual ways. Cutting food into shapes such as stars and animals, numbers and letters will certainly interest young children, and foods which can be eaten with the fingers, such as pizzas, pitta bread and small corn-on-the cobs, are always very popular.

HEALTHY EATING
Healthy eating is all about providing the right kind of food in a balanced way so that the wholesome and natural ingredients can be enjoyed and at the same time provide all the vital nutrients for children's growth and maintenance. Food should be fun, and for children this can be quite easy to do. Encourage them to eat plenty of fresh fruit and vegetables; children are attracted by the bright colours of the many varieties available. Offer a varied selection and introduce exotic fruits as a treat to interest them in new tastes and textures. Most fruits and vegetables can be cut into easy-to-eat sizes which is a good way of serving food to young children. Chunks of apple, and thin sticks of carrot and cucumber are great snack foods for children of all ages.

Try to use unrefined ingredients and food rich in starch and fibre, such as potatoes, rice, pasta and pulses, and limit the intake of refined food, especially sugar. Growing children need plenty of energy, which can be provided by starchy foods, but do not fall into the trap of offering too much fatty or sugary food. Not only will they miss out on other nutrients, but many children can become obese by snacking on chips, crisps, biscuits and sweets. Overweight children with bad eating habits tend to take less exercise and therefore set a pattern which will lead them to all sorts of health problems later on in life.

Children's teeth are at risk from tooth decay, and forbidding sweets at a young age will only make them more attractive. Reduce the damage by limiting sweets to a certain time, such as at the end of a meal, and offer them as a treat, rather than part of everyday eating. Do not use them as a reward to comfort an unhappy child, young children can be very manipulative with tantrums and it is very easy to placate a child with sweets. Avoid giving children fizzy drinks and squashes laden with sugar. Choose fruit juice and dilute it with mineral water, as it is quite high in natural sugar. Choose breakfast cereals with little or no added sugar. Baby foods and drinks do not need sugar added to them.

CHILDREN'S TASTES
Children's tastes often go in phases of likes and dislike, one day a child can be off cheese then suddenly they adore cheese-topped pizzas. They may have a passion for dishes that are not necessarily the healthiest, for example beefburgers and sausages are often favourite foods, so either make your own with very lean meats or buy low fat varieties and grill rather than fry; similarly grill or bake fish fingers. It is also a good idea to cut down on animal sources of fat such as butter, full fat cheeses and red meat.

Very young children rely on milk as their main food for most of their calories. Children under two years need whole milk; between the ages of two and five providing they are eating a good varied diet, they can drink semi-skimmed milk. Home-made milkshakes with no added sugar make nutritious drinks. Small pots of low fat yogurt or fromage frais are easy to eat and are an excellent snack or dessert for small children.

Remember that children's appetites vary greatly, they often prefer smaller meals and snacks throughout the day and can be put off by larger meals. In this book there are plenty of recipe ideas for both main meals and healthy snack foods. The portions are a guideline, as much will depend on the age of the children being fed. Often a ten year old can eat twice as much as a seven year old and as a child becomes a teenager it sometimes seems they are continually hungry.

CHILDREN AND THE FAMILY
With today's busy lifestyles, most children's meals will also be the family's meals too. For mothers at

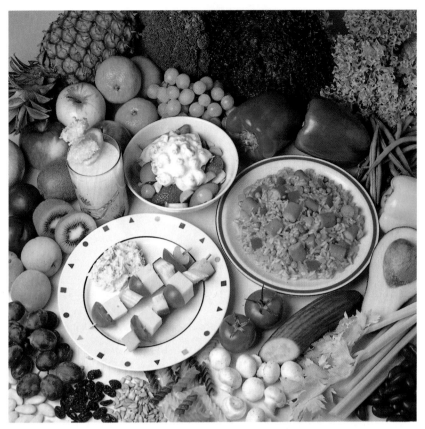

home with young children, the recipes in this book will provide lots of new and attractive ideas. But for working mothers there is rarely enough time to cook children's food separately. It is important that the food chosen for family meals is appealing to everyone, with an emphasis on healthy ingredients. Many of the recipes in the lunches and suppers section can be enjoyed by both children and adults; in the main, children eat smaller versions of adult meals. If we want our children to grow up with good eating habits then it is also important for parents to set an example by eating the right kinds of foods when sharing family meals with their children.

General guidelines apply when shopping for all ages, read the labels on foods to check they are low in fat. Keep a supply of quick cooking low fat foods such as fish fillets and chicken portions in the freezer.

Avoid frying – grill, steam or bake with minimal fat or use a microwave. Use oil or fat sparingly, avoiding blended oils. Choose one that is high in unsaturates such as sunflower or margarine labelled 'high in polyunsaturates'. When a baby or younger child is sharing the family food it is best not to add salt, pepper or spice. These can always be added at the table as can other condiments.

Take advantage of labour saving equipment such as the food processor and microwave oven. Microwave ovens work quickly, enabling you to produce quick snacks, and they cook foods with a minimal amount of water, preventing the unnecessary loss of nutrients from foods such as fresh fruit and vegetables.

A VEGETARIAN IN THE FAMILY

An increasing number of people are eating vegetarian meals, including many children who choose to become vegetarians. A parent whose child chooses to be a vegetarian will need to learn which foods provide protein, such as pulses, milk products and alternatives like tofu made from soya beans. A family diet can be altered to suit a vegetarian child and remain very healthy, with the emphasis on wholefoods, grains and seeds. Vegetable burgers and patties, vegetarian sausages and grills are not just for vegetarians, they add variety to the diet and can be enjoyed by the whole family. There are several recipes throughout the book which do not use meat, they are still attractive, fun and nutritious and appeal to everyone.

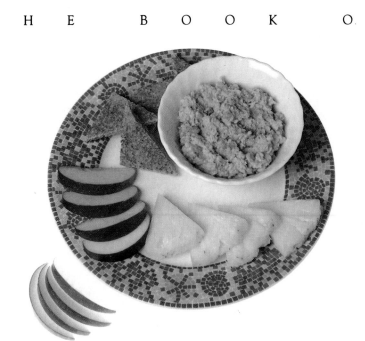

BREAKFAST DIP

115 g (4 oz/½ cup) crunchy peanut butter
2 tablespoons sesame seeds
6 tablespoons low fat natural yogurt
2 thick slices bread
2 dessert apples
½ small pineapple

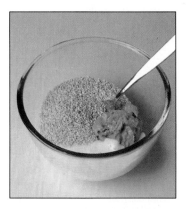

Put the peanut butter, sesame seeds and yogurt into a bowl and mix together until they are well blended.

Toast the slices of bread on each side, remove the crusts and cut each slice into 8 triangles.

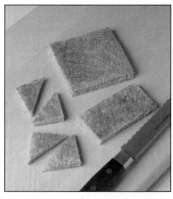

Quarter the apples, remove the cores and cut each piece into 3 slices. Cut the skin off the pineapple and discard. Cut the pineapple into neat pieces. Serve the dip with the toast and fruit.

Serves 4-6.

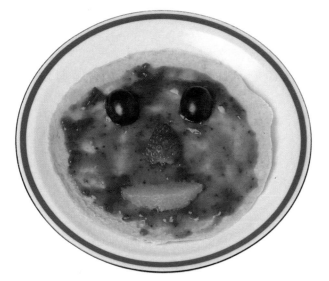

FRUITY PANCAKE FACES

55 g (2 oz/½ cup) wholemeal flour
55 g (2 oz/½ cup) plain flour
2 eggs, beaten
300 ml (10 fl oz/1¼ cups) milk
1 orange
4 strawberries
8 grapes
4 tablespoons reduced-sugar jam
25 g (1 oz/6 teaspoons) butter

Put the flours into a bowl, make a well in the centre, add the eggs and milk and whisk together to form a smooth batter.

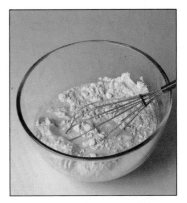

Allow the batter to stand while preparing the fruit. Peel and segment the orange and halve the strawberries and grapes; remove the pips from the grapes. Put the jam into a small saucepan and warm gently to soften. To make the pancakes, heat a small frying pan, about 12.5 cm (5 in) in diameter, over a medium-high heat. Melt a very small knob of butter in the pan (you need just enough to coat the surface).

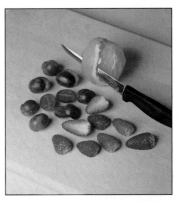

Pour in enough batter to thickly cover the base of the pan. Cook until the batter is no longer runny and the underside is lightly browned. Turn the pancake over and cook for about 30-45 seconds. Slide the pancake onto a plate. To serve, spread a spoonful of jam over each one, place a segment of orange for the 'mouth', half a strawberry for the 'nose' and grape halves for 'eyes'.

Makes 8 pancakes.

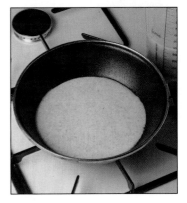

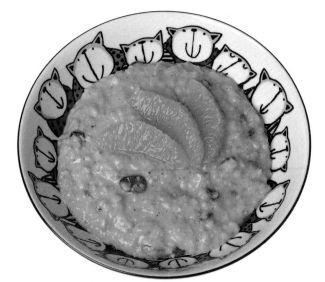

——— BREAKFAST SURPRISE ———

2 large oranges
115 g (4 oz/1⅓ cups) quick-cook porridge oats
450 ml (16 fl oz/2 cups) milk
55 g (2 oz/⅓ cup) raisins or sultanas
1 tablespoon clear honey

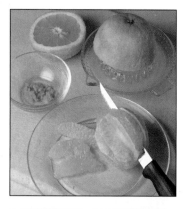

Grate the rind from one of the oranges and squeeze out the juice. Remove the skin and pith from the remaining orange and cut into segments; set aside.

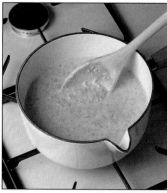

Put the orange rind, juice, oats and milk into a saucepan, bring slowly to the boil, stirring all the time, and then cook over a low heat for 1 minute.

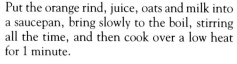
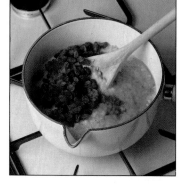

Stir in the raisins or sultanas with the honey. Divide between 4 serving bowls and decorate each portion with some of the orange segments. Serve at once.

Serves 4.

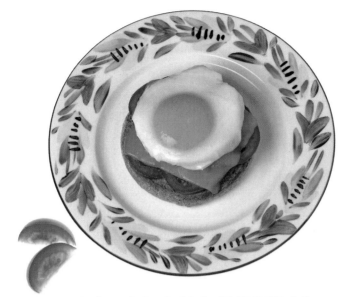

SAVOURY MUFFINS

2 wholemeal muffins
sunflower margarine
yeast extract (optional)
2 large tomatoes, sliced
4 slices Cheddar or Edam cheese
4 eggs

Cut the muffins in half, lightly toast, then spread with a little margarine and yeast extract, if using.

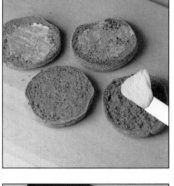

Divide the tomato slices between the muffins and place a slice of cheese on top. Place under a hot grill until just beginning to melt.

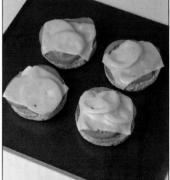

Meanwhile pour about 2.5 cm (1 in) water into a large frying pan and bring to simmering point. Break each egg into the water and poach over a medium heat until the eggs are cooked. Lift out with a slotted spoon and place an egg on each muffin. Serve at once.

Serves 4.

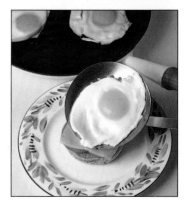

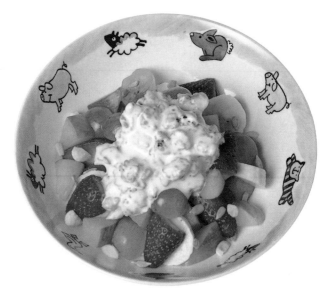

— FRUITY MORNING STARTER —

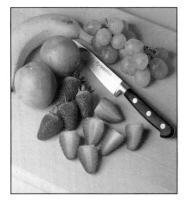

115 g (4 oz) strawberries
115 g (4 oz) grapes
1 peach or nectarine or 2 plums
1 banana
2 tablespoons almonds, coarsely chopped
1 tablespoon sunflower seeds
5 tablespoons natural yogurt
2 teaspoons clear honey
3 tablespoons crunchy oat cereal

Wash, hull and halve the strawberries. Halve grapes and remove the pips. Dice the peach and slice the banana. Put the fruit into a bowl and mix together.

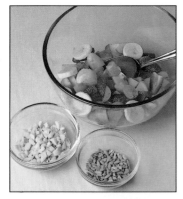

Add the almonds and sunflower seeds to the fruits and mix lightly together, then divide between 4 serving dishes.

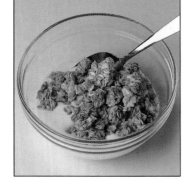

Mix the yogurt with the honey and stir in the cereal, then spoon over the fruit and serve.

Serves 4.

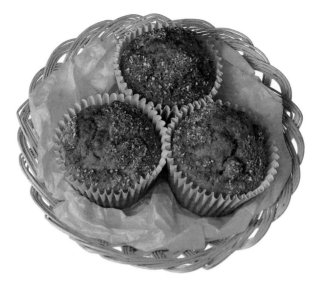

—— BANANA MUFFINS ——

115 g (4 oz/1 cup) plain flour
115 g (4 oz/1 cup) wholemeal flour
3 teaspoons baking powder
55 g (2 oz/½ cup) medium oatmeal
55 g (2 oz/⅓ cup) light soft brown sugar
55 g (2oz/½ cup) walnuts, chopped
2 eggs
55 ml (2 fl oz/¼ cup) clear honey
150 ml (5 fl oz/⅔ cup) milk
3 tablespoons sunflower oil
few drops vanilla essence
2 ripe bananas
TO FINISH:
2 teaspoons oatmeal
2 teaspoons demerara sugar

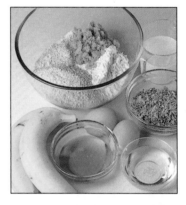

Preheat oven to 200C (400F/Gas 6). Sift the flours and baking powder into a bowl, then add the bran remaining in the sieve. Stir in the oatmeal, sugar and nuts. Whisk together the eggs, honey, milk, oil and vanilla essence, add to the dry ingredients and stir together. Roughly mash the bananas and stir into the mixture.

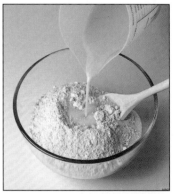

Divide the mixture between 12 paper cases placed in a deep-holed muffin or tartlet tin. Mix the 2 teaspoons oatmeal and demerara sugar together and scatter over the top of the muffins. Bake in the oven for 20-25 minutes until golden.

Makes 12.

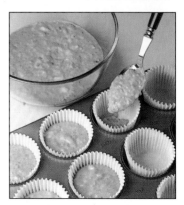

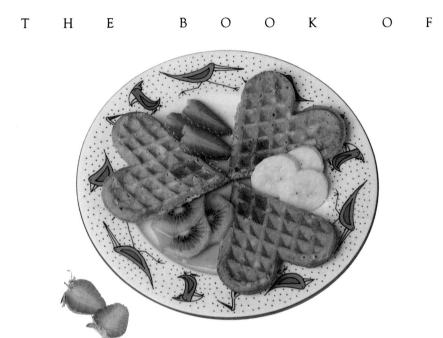

OAT WAFFLES

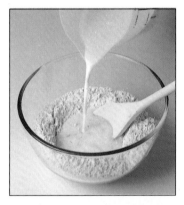

115 g (4 oz/1 cup) plain flour
115 g (4 oz/1 cup) wholemeal flour
55 g (2 oz/²⁄₃ cup) rolled oats
55 g (2 oz/¹⁄₃ cup) light soft brown sugar
2 teaspoons baking powder
½ teaspoon salt
2 eggs
350 ml (12 fl oz/1½ cups) milk
2 tablespoons sunflower oil
oil for cooking

Put flours, oats, sugar, baking powder and salt into a bowl. Beat together the eggs, milk and oil; add to bowl.

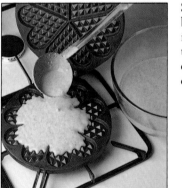

Stir the ingredients together until well blended, using a wooden spoon. Heat a waffle iron according to the manufacturer's instructions. Brush the surface with a little oil. Ladle enough batter onto the preheated surface to cover about two-thirds of it.

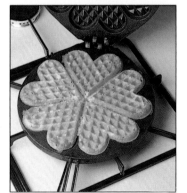

Close the lid and cook the waffles on a medium heat for about 2 minutes each side until crisp and golden. Serve the waffles at once, topped with thick yogurt or maple syrup and pieces of fruit or a fruit purée.

Makes 25-30.

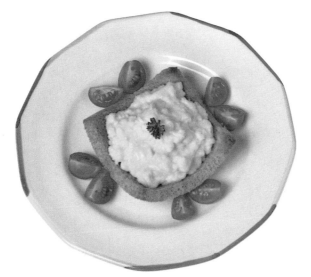

– SCRAMBLED EGG SCRUNCHIES –

55 g (2 oz/¼ cup) butter
4 large slices bread, crusts removed
4 eggs
2 tablespoons milk
salt and pepper
25 g (1 oz/¼ cup) grated Cheddar cheese
tomato wedges and parsley sprigs, to garnish

Preheat oven to 200C (400F/Gas 6). Melt half the butter and brush both sides of each bread slice with the melted butter.

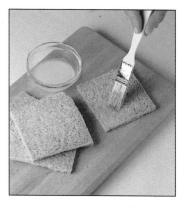

Line 4 individual 7.5 cm (3 in) flan tins with the bread slices, pressing them down well in the centre but leaving the corners pointing up. Bake in the oven for 15-20 minutes until crisp and golden.

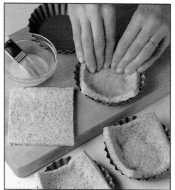

About 5 minutes before the bread cases are ready, beat the eggs and milk together and stir in the seasoning and cheese. Melt the remaining butter in a saucepan and pour in the egg mixture. Cook over a gentle heat, stirring all the time until the eggs are just set but still creamy. Remove from the heat, spoon into the bread cases and serve immediately. Garnish with wedges of tomato and parsley sprigs.

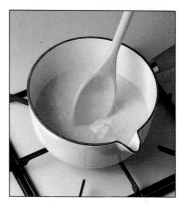

Serves 4.

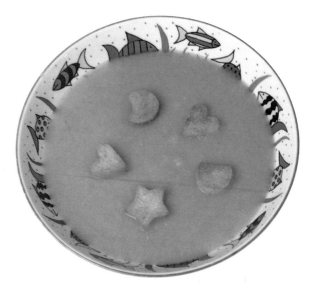

SUNSHINE SOUP

15 g (½ oz/3 teaspoons) butter or margarine
1 small onion, finely chopped
350 g (12 oz) carrots, chopped
25 g (1 oz/2 tablespoons) split red lentils
550 ml (20 fl oz/2½ cups) vegetable stock
juice 1 small orange
CROÛTONS:
2 slices bread
sunflower oil for frying

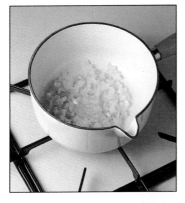

Melt the butter in a saucepan, add the onion and cook gently until soft.

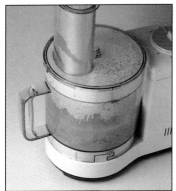

Add the carrots and lentils, stir together, then pour in the stock. Bring to the boil, then simmer for 15-20 minutes until the carrots are tender. Purée in a blender or food processor until very smooth.

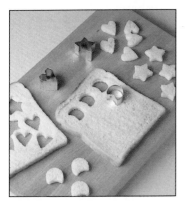

Return the mixture to the pan and reheat, then stir in the orange juice. Keep warm. To make croûtons, stamp out some attractive shapes from the bread using small biscuit cutters. Heat a little oil in a frying pan and cook the bread shapes until golden. Drain on absorbent kitchen paper and serve as a garnish with the soup.

Serves 4-5.

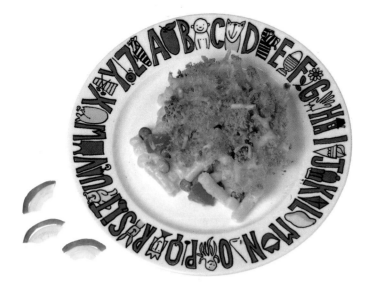

– RAINBOW MACARONI CHEESE –

115 g (4 oz/¾ cup) macaroni
15 g (½ oz/6 teaspoons) plain flour
15 g (½ oz/3 teaspoons) butter
300 ml (10 fl oz/1¼ cups) milk
salt and pepper
55 g (2 oz) frozen peas
55 g (2 oz) frozen sweetcorn
1 tomato, diced
85 g (3 oz/¾ cup) grated Gouda or Edam cheese
25 g (1 oz/½ cup) wholemeal breadcrumbs

Half-fill a saucepan with water and bring to the boil. Add 1 teaspoon salt, then stir in the macaroni and cook for 7 minutes until tender. Drain.

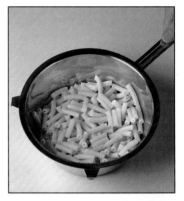

Put the flour, butter and milk into a medium saucepan and cook over a medium heat, whisking all the time until thickened. Season with a little salt and pepper, turn the heat to low and add the peas, sweetcorn, diced tomato and 55 g (2 oz/½ cup) of the cheese. Stir and cook for 2 minutes.

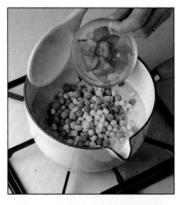

Mix the macaroni into the sauce and heat through. Spoon the mixture into 4 small ovenproof dishes or 1 large one. Mix the breadcrumbs with the remaining cheese and sprinkle on top. Place under a hot grill for 3-4 minutes to brown. Serve immediately.

Serves 4.

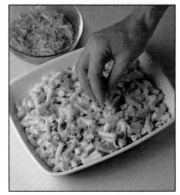

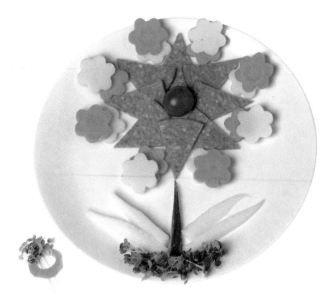

———CHILDREN'S ANTIPASTO———

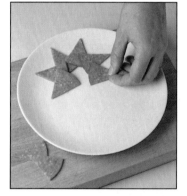

4 slices mild salami or ham sausage
2 cherry tomatoes
115 g (4 oz) piece mild cheese or Edam cheese slices
2 large carrots, sliced
5 cm (2 in) piece cucumber
a little cress, washed

Cut each slice of salami into 4 and divide between 2 plates, arranging it in a circle with the points facing out. Place a tomato in the middle of each.

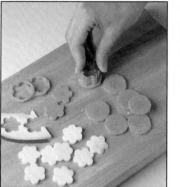

Cut the cheese into slices, then using a small petal-shaped cutter, cut out shapes (the spare bits can be grated and used for a sauce). Cut out petals from the slices of carrot and arrange with the cheese around the edge of the plate to look like flower petals.

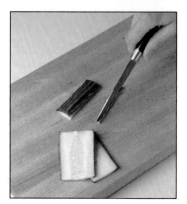

Cut a long slice of cucumber, then cut 2 thin strips to resemble 'stalks' for the flowers. Cut long slices from the rest of the cucumber and shape them to look like 'leaves'; place 4 on each flower. Snip the cress and arrange on the plate to look like 'grass'.

Serves 2.

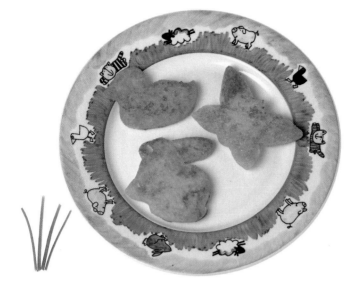

——— ANIMAL EGGY BREADS ———

6 slices bread
1 large egg
3 tablespoons milk
45 g (1½ oz/9 teaspoons) butter

Cut the bread into animal shapes using a variety of biscuit cutters.

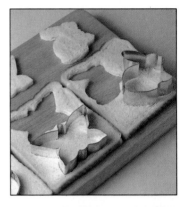

Beat the egg and milk together and put into a shallow dish.

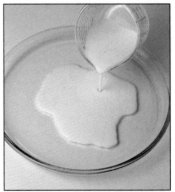

Melt the butter in a large frying pan. Dip the bread shapes in the egg mixture, coating each side, then place in the frying pan and cook on each side until golden. Serve at once.

Makes about 12 pieces.

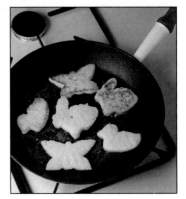

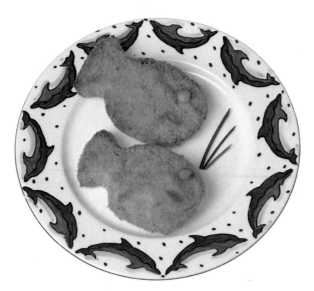

FUN FISH CAKES

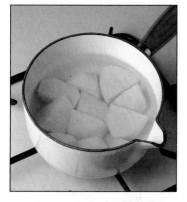

225 g (8 oz) potatoes, peeled
25 g (1 oz/6 teaspoons) butter
1 egg yolk
1 tablespoon chopped chives
200 g (7 oz) can tuna in brine, drained
1 egg, beaten
85 g (3 oz/¾ cup) dry golden breadcrumbs
6 peas
1 small tomato
chives, to garnish

Preheat oven to 200C (400F/Gas 6). Cut the potatoes into even pieces, put into a pan of water and boil until just tender.

Drain the potatoes, return to pan and dry over a low heat for a few moments. Add the butter and egg yolk and mash together. Stir in the chives and tuna. Divide the mixture into 6 equal portions and, with floured hands, shape into flat pear shapes. Shape the thinner end of the cakes to form a 'V' shape like the tail of a fish.

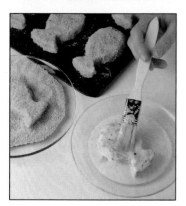

Put the beaten egg into a shallow dish. Place the fish cakes in the egg and brush with egg. Coat in breadcrumbs, then place on a greased baking sheet. Brush with a little oil and bake for 20-25 minutes until crisp and golden. To serve, place a pea on each fish for an 'eye' and add a small sliver of tomato for the mouth. Garnish with chives and serve hot.

Makes 6.

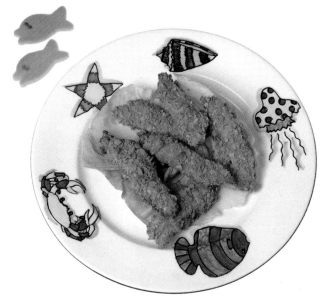

FISH FLIPS

3 plaice or flounder fillets, weighing about 300 g
  (10 oz), skinned
2 tablespoons plain flour
salt and pepper
1 egg, beaten
85 g (3 oz/3 cups) cornflakes, crushed
lettuce leaves, to serve

Preheat oven to 190C (375F/Gas 5). Grease
2 baking sheets with oil. Cut the plaice or
flounder fillets into strips about 1 cm
(½ in) wide.

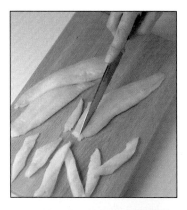

Dust the strips in flour which has been
seasoned with salt and pepper, then dip into
the beaten egg.

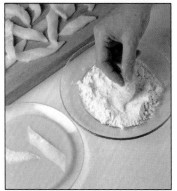

Coat the strips in the crushed cornflakes,
then place on the baking sheets. Bake in the
oven for 15 minutes until the coating is crisp.
Serve about 6 strips per serving, on a bed of
lettuce leaves.

Serves 4.

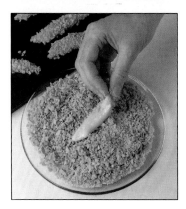

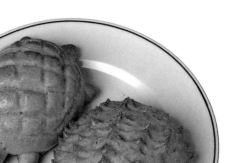

——ANIMAL BREAD ROLLS——

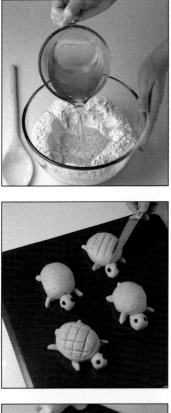

225 g (8 oz/2 cups) wholemeal flour
225 g (8 oz/2 cups) strong white flour
1 sachet easy blend dried yeast
pinch salt
1 tablespoon vegetable oil
2 teaspoons clear honey
300 ml (10 fl oz/1¼ cups) tepid water
currants, to decorate
1 egg, beaten

Grease 2 baking sheets. In a large bowl, mix the flours, yeast and salt together. Make a well in the centre. Mix the oil with honey and water, then pour into the well.

Mix to form a firm dough. Turn the dough onto a floured surface and knead well, then divide into 8 pieces. From 4 pieces, take a small piece large enough to form a tail and 4 feet and a slightly larger one for the head. Shape the large piece into a round shape and flatten slightly. Shape and attach the very small pieces to look like feet and a tail, then attach the larger piece for the head and place 2 currants in position for the 'eyes'. Transfer to a baking sheet. With a sharp knife, mark the top of the body in a criss-cross pattern, to look like a tortoise.

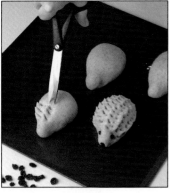

With the remaining 4 pieces of dough, shape each into an oval and shape one end to a point. Transfer to a baking sheet. Using sharp scissors, snip the top to look like prickles on a hedgehog and insert currants for 'eyes' and 'nose'. Leave in a warm place for 30 minutes until almost doubled in size. Preheat the oven to 230C (450F/Gas 8). Brush the animals with beaten egg. Bake for 15-20 minutes until cooked through and golden.

Makes 8.

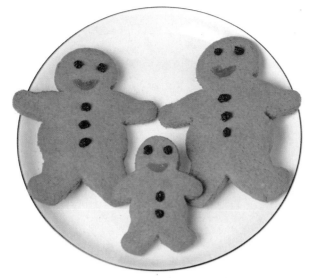

———GINGERBREAD FRIENDS———

225 g (8 oz/1¾ cups) wholemeal flour
1 teaspoon bicarbonate of soda
1 teaspoon ground cinnamon
1 teaspoon ground ginger
85 g (3 oz/⅓ cup) margarine
115 g (4 oz/¾ cup) light soft brown sugar
2 tablespoons golden syrup
3 teaspoons orange juice
currants and glacé cherry, to decorate

Preheat oven to 170C (325F/Gas 3). Grease 2 baking sheets. Place the flour in a mixing bowl, then sift on the bircarbonate of soda and spices.

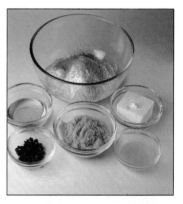

Put the margarine, sugar and syrup in a pan and heat gently, stirring until melted. Cool, then pour onto the flour with the orange juice and mix to a firm dough.

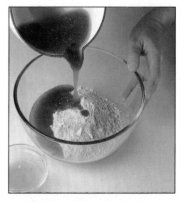

Turn onto a floured surface and roll out to about 0.5cm (¼ in) thick. Using gingerbread men and women cutters, cut out figures and place them on the baking sheets. Decorate with currants and slivers of glacé cherry. Bake in the oven for 15 minutes until firm. Cool slightly, then transfer to a wire rack to cool completely. Store in an airtight tin.

Makes 8-10.

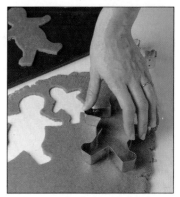

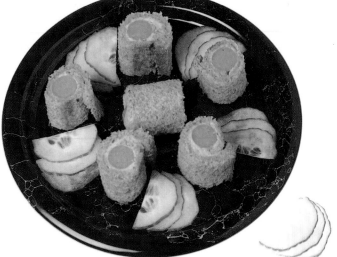

— SAUSAGE WHEELS —

8 slices wholemeal bread, crusts removed
4 tablespoons medium fat soft cheese
2 tablespoons tomato ketchup (sauce)
8 frankfurters
25 g (1 oz/6 teaspoons) butter, melted
cucumber slices, to garnish

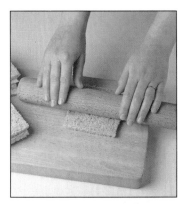

Preheat oven to 190C (375F/Gas 5). Roll the slices of bread thinly with a rolling pin.

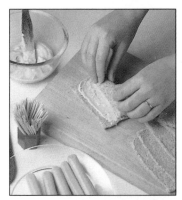

Mix the cheese and tomato ketchup (sauce) together and spread over each slice of bread. Place a frankfurter at one end of the bread, then roll up and secure each with 2 wooden cocktail sticks.

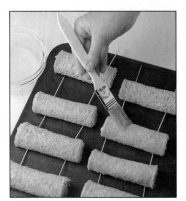

Place on a baking sheet and brush with melted butter. Bake in the oven for 15 minutes until crisp. Remove the cocktail sticks and cut each roll into 3 before serving, garnished with cucumber slices.

Makes 24.

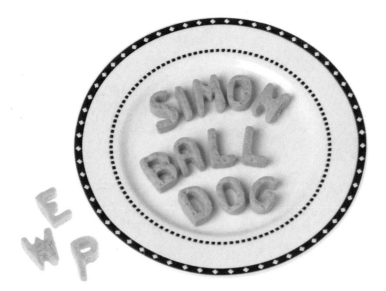

——————— ALPHABET BISCUITS ———————

55 g (2 oz/3 tablespoons) smooth peanut butter
55 g (2 oz/¼ cup) sunflower margarine
55 g (2 oz/¼ cup) light muscovado sugar
1 egg, beaten
175 g (6 oz/1½ cups) plain flour

Preheat oven to 180C (350F/Gas 4). Grease 2 or 3 baking sheets. Put the peanut butter and margarine into a bowl, add the sugar and beat until creamy.

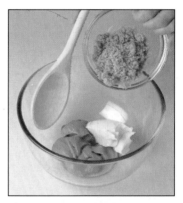

Beat in the egg, then sift in the flour and mix together for form a dough. Turn onto a floured surface and knead lightly.

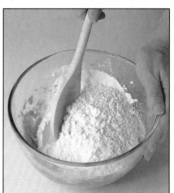

Roll out the dough to about 0.5 cm (¼ in) thick. Using small alphabet cutters, stamp out letters and place them on the prepared baking sheets. Gather up the trimmings and re-roll, then cut out as many letters as possible. Bake the biscuits in the oven for 10-12 minutes. Cool on a wire rack.

Makes approximately 100 small letters.

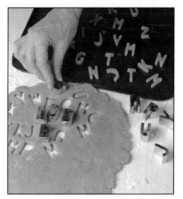

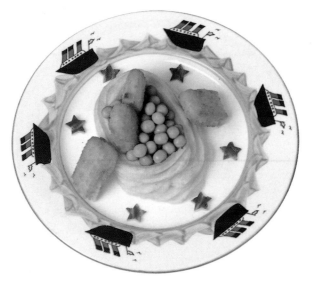

POTATO RAFTS

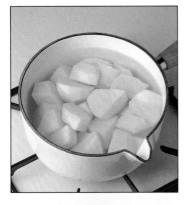

450 g (1 lb) potatoes, peeled
salt
25 g (1 oz/6 teaspoons) butter
115 g (4 oz) frozen peas
8 fish fingers
cucumber stars, to garnish (optional)

Cut the potatoes into even pieces, put into a pan of salted water and boil until tender.

Drain the potatoes, return to pan and dry over a low heat for a few moments. Add the butter and mash until very smooth. Spoon into a piping bag fitted with a large star nozzle and pipe 4 boat-shaped nests of potato onto a baking sheet.

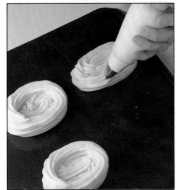

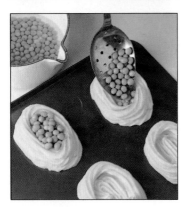

Grill the boats until golden and cook the fish fingers under the grill untill browned and cooked through. Cook the peas following packet instructions. To assemble, fill the boats with peas. Halve the fish fingers and place 2 halves in the middle of each boat to look like 'sails' and place the remainder on the sides to look like 'oars'.

Serves 4.

Variation: Replace peas with baked beans and fish fingers with cooked sausages.

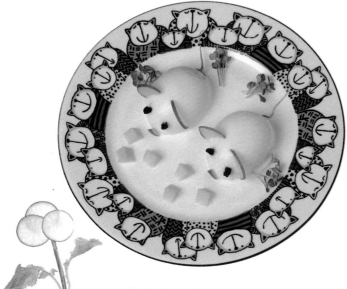

CHEESY MICE

4 eggs, hard-boiled and shelled
25 g (1 oz/¼ cup) finely grated Cheddar cheese
25 g (1 oz/6 teaspoons) low fat soft cheese
8 radishes
16 currants
55 g (2 oz) Edam cheese, cut into small chunks
salad cress

Carefully halve the eggs lengthways and scoop out the yolks into a bowl.

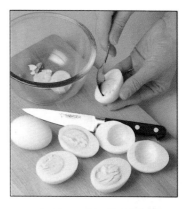

Add the grated cheese and low fat cheese and mix together until smooth. Spoon into the egg whites and smooth the surface.

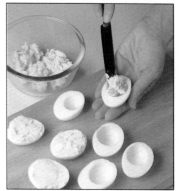

To assemble each mouse, cut slits at the pointed end of the eggs, and insert small slices of radish for 'ears', currants for 'eyes', and small pieces of radish for a 'nose'. Attach the radish roots for 'tails'. Place the egg mice on serving plates and arrange small chunks of cheese in front and little bunches of salad cress on each plate.

Serves 4.

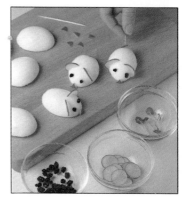

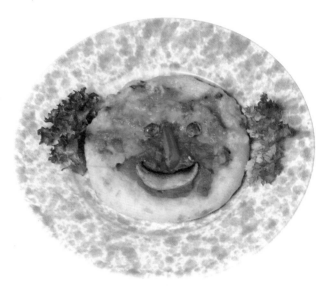

FUNNY FACE PIZZAS

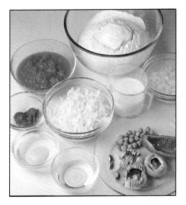

2 teaspoons oil
½ small onion
200 g (7 oz) can chopped tomatoes
3 teaspoons tomato purée (paste)
350 g (12 oz/3 cups) self-raising flour
1 teaspoon salt
85 g (3 oz/⅓ cup) sunflower margarine
115 g (4 oz/1 cup) grated mild Cheddar cheese
1 egg
150 ml (5 fl oz/⅔ cup) milk
24 peas
3 large button mushrooms
small piece red, orange or yellow pepper (capsicum)
lollo rosso lettuce, to garnish

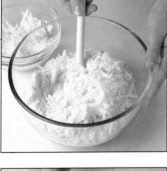

Heat oil in a small pan, add the onion and cook until soft. Stir in the tomatoes and purée (paste) and cook over medium heat for 10 minutes until thickened. Preheat oven to 200C (400F/Gas 6). Grease 2 baking sheets. Sift flour and salt into a bowl, rub in margarine, then stir in half the cheese. Beat the egg with the milk; add to the bowl and mix to form a smooth ball of dough. Divide dough into 12 pieces and roll out each one to 7.5 cm (3 in) round and place 6 on each of the baking sheets.

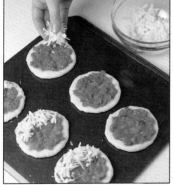

Divide the tomato sauce between the rounds. Place the remaining grated cheese on one edge to resemble 'hair'. Add the peas to look like 'eyes'. Slice the mushrooms, discard the stalks and place a slice on each pizza to resemble a 'mouth'. Cut the pepper (capsicum) into strips and arrange on each pizza to look like a 'nose'. Bake the pizzas in the oven for 12-15 minutes until the edges are golden. Garnish with red lollo rosso lettuce to resemble 'hair'.

Makes 12.

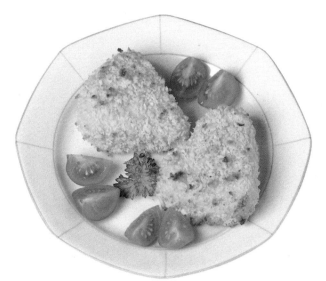

SURPRISE TRIANGLES

6 heaped tablespoons cooked mashed potato
6 processed cheese triangles
1 egg, beaten
55 g (2 oz/1 cup) fresh breadcrumbs
25 g (1 oz/¼ cup) peanuts, very finely chopped
12 cherry tomatoes, cut into wedges
parsley sprigs, to garnish

Preheat oven to 200C (400F/Gas 6). Place 1 tablespoon potato on a floured surface and spread out to about 0.5 cm (¼ in) thick. Place a cheese triangle in the centre.

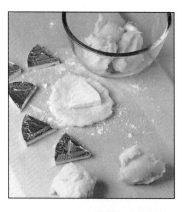

Mould the potato around the cheese, keeping a neat triangular shape. Repeat with the rest of the potato and cheese.

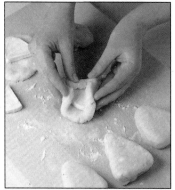

Place each triangle in beaten egg and brush with egg, then coat in the breadcrumbs mixed with the chopped peanuts. Place on a greased baking sheet and bake in the oven for 15 minutes until crisp. Serve with cherry tomatoes and garnish with parsley sprigs.

Makes 6.

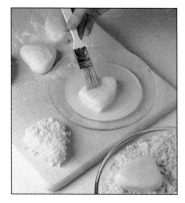

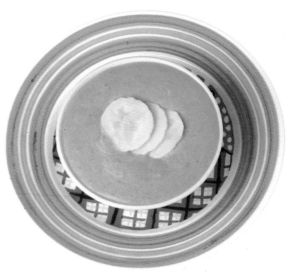

—CHOCOLATE BANANA WHIP—

300 ml (10 fl oz/1¼ cups) milk
55 g (2 oz) milk chocolate drops
9 teaspoons cornflour
25 g (1 oz/6 teaspoons) sugar
3 small bananas
150 ml (5 fl oz/⅔ cup) whipping cream

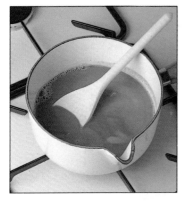

Put all but 2 tablespoons of the milk and the chocolate drops in a saucepan and heat gently until the chocolate melts, stirring frequently with a wooden spoon.

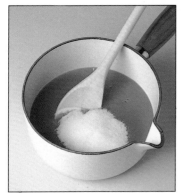

Put the cornflour into a bowl, add the reserved milk and blend together, then whisk in the rest of the chocolate milk. Return to the saucepan and bring to the boil, stirring. Reduce heat and simmer for 1 minute, until thickened. Remove from the heat and stir in the sugar. Cover with a piece of greaseproof paper and set aside to cool.

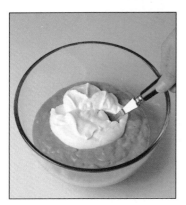

Mash 2 of the bananas and fold into the cold chocolate custard. Whip the cream until softly peaking, then fold into the mixture. Spoon into serving dishes and refrigerate until needed. Decorate with slices of remaining banana. (This dessert is best eaten the day it is made.)

Serves 4-6.

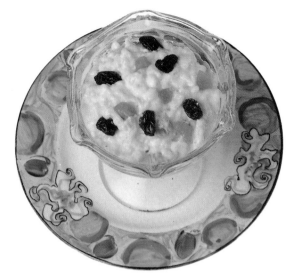

─── SPECIAL RICE PUDDING ───

55 g (2 oz/¼ cup) short-grain rice
550 ml (20 fl oz/2½ cups) milk
2 tablespoons sugar
few drops vanilla essence
55 g (2 oz) ready-to-eat dried apricots, chopped
4 tablespoons natural yogurt or apricot flavoured
   yogurt
1 tablespoon each raisins and chopped ready-to-eat
   dried apricots, to decorate

Put the rice into a saucepan, add the milk and bring slowly to the boil. Lower the heat and simmer gently for 40 minutes, stirring occasionally.

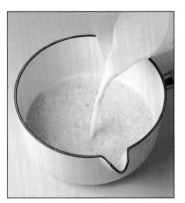

Stir in the sugar, vanilla essence and chopped apricots, then turn the mixture into a bowl and leave to cool.

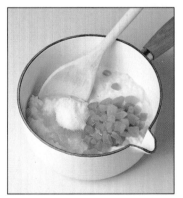

Fold in the yogurt and chill until needed. Spoon into serving glasses and decorate with raisins and chopped apricots.

Serves 4-6.

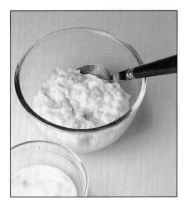

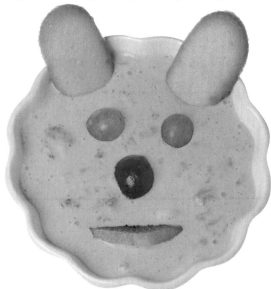

——————— TEDDY BEAR FOOL ———————

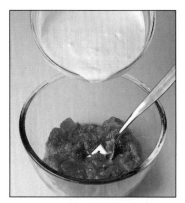

225 g (8 oz) strawberries, washed and hulled
300 ml (10 fl oz/1¼ cups) thick Greek yogurt
2-3 teaspoons clear honey
8 thin finger biscuits
8 seedless grapes
2 glacé cherries, halved
2 slices kiwi fruit, halved

In a bowl, mash the strawberries slightly (do not make them completely smooth).

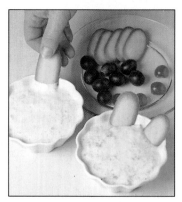

Whisk the yogurt with the honey until smooth and creamy. Add to the mashed strawberries and mix well. Divide the mixture between 4 serving dishes. Decorate by placing the biscuits in position to resemble the 'ears'.

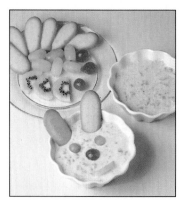

Position the seedless grapes for 'eyes', a cherry half for the 'nose' and finally press one halved slice of kiwi fruit into each fool to resemble a 'mouth'.

Serves 4.

Variation: Cook 115 g (4 oz) ready-to-eat dried apricots until soft; purée and mix into the yogurt. Or mash 2 small, ripe bananas and add to the yogurt.

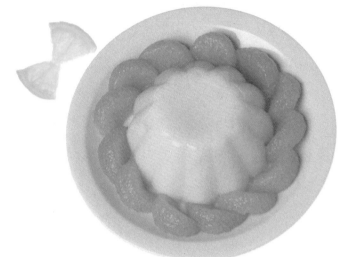

JELLY WOBBLES

4 oranges
55 g (2 oz/¼ cup) sugar
150 ml (5 fl oz/⅔ cup) water
15 g (½ oz/5 teaspoons) powdered gelatine
150 ml (5 fl oz/⅔ cup) natural yogurt
312 g (11 oz) can mandarin segments in natural juice,
   drained

Using a vegetable peeler, pare the rind from 2 oranges and put into a saucepan with the sugar and water. Bring to the boil and simmer until the sugar has dissolved. Allow to stand for a few minutes. Squeeze the juice from all of the oranges and reserve.

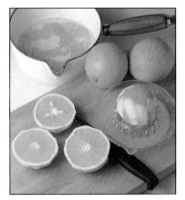

Strain the sugar, water and orange rind liquid into a bowl. Measure 3 tablespoons cold water into a small heatproof bowl, sprinkle over the gelatine and leave for a few minutes to become spongy. Stand bowl in a pan with a little simmering water until the gelatine has dissolved, then add to the strained liquid. Allow to cool, then add the orange juice and refrigerate until beginning to set.

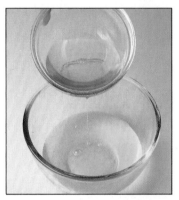

Whisk in the yogurt and pour into 4 or 5 small moulds. Return to the refrigerator for 2-3 hours to set. To serve, turn out into small dishes and decorate each portion with mandarin orange segments.

Serves 4-5.

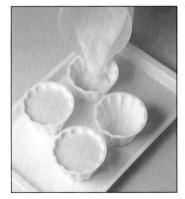

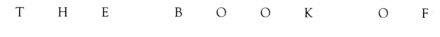

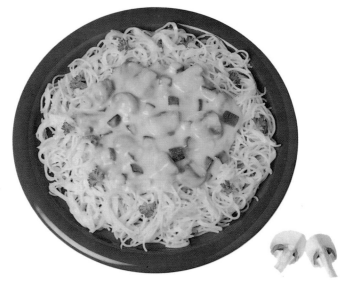

VERMICELLI NESTS

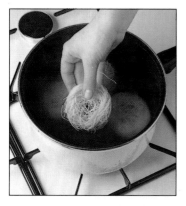

115 g (4 oz) vermicelli
25 g (1 oz/6 teaspoons) butter
55 g (2 oz) onion, chopped
1 courgette (zucchini), diced
175 g (6 oz) button mushrooms, quartered
15 g (½ oz/6 teaspoons) plain flour
250 ml (8 fl oz/1 cup) milk
pinch grated nutmeg
salt and pepper
55 g (2 oz/½ cup) grated Cheddar cheese
chopped parsley, to garnish

Put the vermicelli into a large pan of salted boiling water and cook for about 6 minutes until tender.

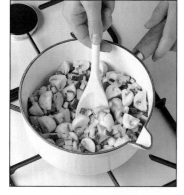

Meanwhile melt the butter in a saucepan, add the onion, courgette (zucchini) and mushrooms and cook for 3-4 minutes until soft. Stir in the flour.

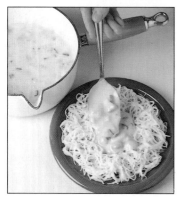

Gradually add the milk, return to the heat and simmer for 2 minutes, stirring all the time. Season with the nutmeg and salt and pepper. Stir in the cheese and heat gently until melted. Drain the vermicelli and divide between 4 plates. Make a hollow in the centres and spoon in the vegetable sauce. Garnish with chopped parsley and serve hot.

Serves 4.

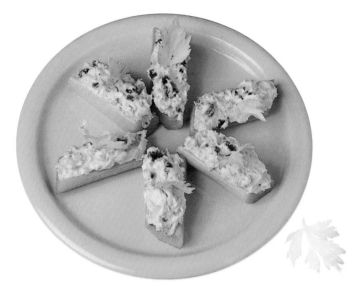

——NUTTY CELERY BOATS——

½ head celery
115 g (4 oz/½ cup) low fat cream cheese
55 g (2 oz/½ cup) finely grated Cheddar cheese
55 g (2 oz/3 tablespoons) crunchy peanut butter
25 g (1 oz/¼ cup) raisins, chopped
55 g (2oz/⅓ cup) chopped peanuts
2 tablespoons fromage frais or natural yogurt
celery leaves, to garnish

Wash the celery and cut the sticks into 5 cm (2 in) lengths.

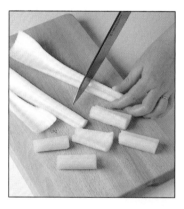

Put all the remaining ingredients, except the garnish, into a bowl and beat together until well blended.

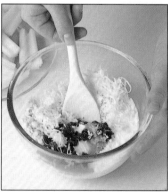

Spread the filling into the celery pieces, mounding it up slightly, and garnish with celery leaves.

Serves 4.

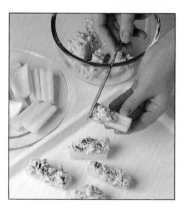

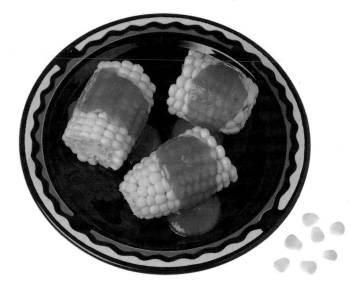

—DEVILLED CORN-ON-THE-COB—

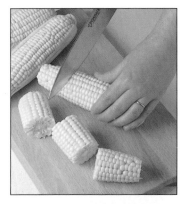

4 corn-on-the cob
85 g (3 oz/⅓ cup) butter
3 tablespoons tomato ketchup (sauce)
2 teaspoons Worcestershire sauce

Remove the husks and silky threads from the corn and with a sturdy knife cut each cob into 3 pieces. Bring a large pan of water to the boil, add the corn and boil for 6-8 minutes, until tender.

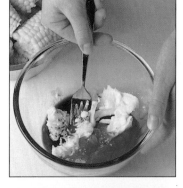

Meanwhile, put the butter into a bowl and mash to soften. Add the tomato ketchup (sauce) and Worcestershire sauce and beat together until well blended.

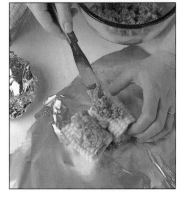

Drain the corn and spread each piece with the butter mixture. Put 2 pieces onto a piece of foil and wrap to form into a tight parcel; repeat with the rest of the corn. Place under a hot grill for 5 minutes. To serve, lift the corn onto a plate and pour over the devilled butter from the foil.

Serves 4-6.

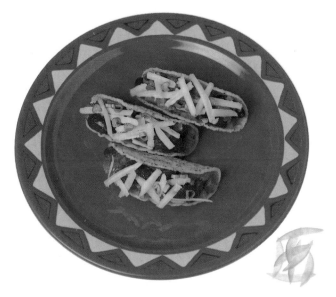

MINI TACOS

1 tablespoon sunflower oil
1 small onion, finely chopped
3 tomatoes, skinned and diced
½ green pepper (capsicum), seeded and chopped
1 tablespoon tomato purée (paste)
½ teaspoon chilli sauce (optional)
200 g (7 oz) can red kidney beans, rinsed and drained
12 mini tacos
55 g (2 oz/½ cup) grated Cheddar cheese
3 spring onions, chopped

Preheat oven to 180C (350F/Gas 4). Heat the oil in a medium saucepan, add the onion and cook until soft.

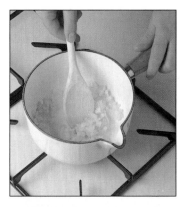

Add the tomatoes, green pepper (capsicum), tomato purée (paste) and chilli sauce (if using) and red kidney beans and simmer for about 7-8 minutes until the mixture is soft.

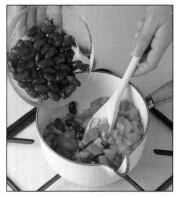

Meanwhile, put the taco shells onto a baking sheet and place in the oven for 3-4 minutes. Divide the filling between the shells, then top with grated cheese and a little chopped spring onion.

Serves 3-4.

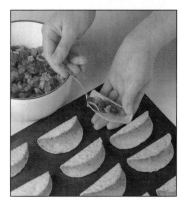

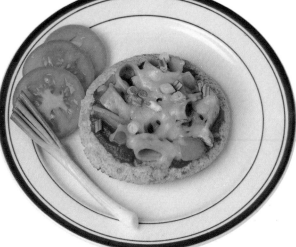

PITTA PIZZAS

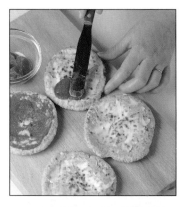

4 small wholemeal pitta breads
a little sunflower margarine
4 teaspoons tomato purée (paste)
2 large tomatoes, chopped
4 large slices ham or garlic sausage
pinch mixed herbs
55 g (2 oz/½ cup) grated Cheddar cheese
3 spring onions, chopped

Spread a little sunflower margarine over one side of each pitta bread. Spread a teaspoon of tomato purée (paste) on top.

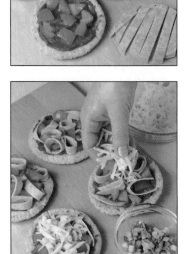

Divide the chopped tomatoes between the pittas. Cut the slices of ham or garlic sausage into strips and arrange on top. Sprinkle with a pinch of herbs.

Scatter over the cheese and spring onions. Place under a hot grill for 3-5 minutes until heated through, and the cheese has melted.

Serves 4.

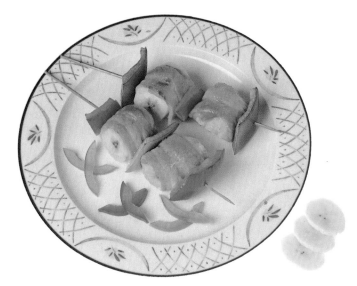

— BANANA & BACON ROLLS —

4 large bananas (slightly under-ripe)
8 very lean bacon rashers, halved
1 red pepper (capsicum), seeded and cut into pieces
1 green pepper (capsicum), seeded and cut into pieces
1 tablespoon sunflower oil
1 tablespoon soy sauce
1 teaspoon clear honey

Peel the bananas and cut each into 4 pieces. Wrap each piece of banana in a halved bacon rasher.

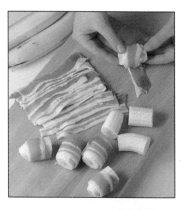

Thread the bacon rolls onto bamboo skewers with the peppers.

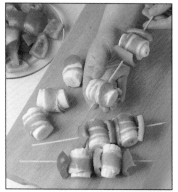

Mix the oil, soy sauce and honey together and brush over the kebabs. Place under a hot grill, turning them during cooking and brushing them with the oil mixture, until the bacon is golden.

Serves 4.

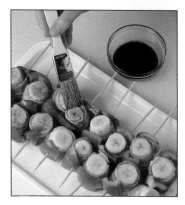

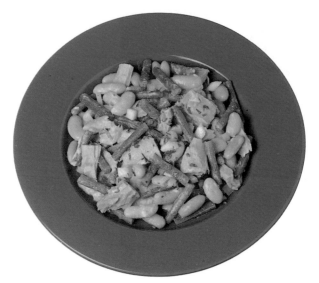

——TUNA & BEAN SALAD——

175 g (6 oz) French green beans
1 tablespoon finely chopped onion
400 g (14 oz) can cannellini beans, drained
200 g (7 oz) can tuna in brine, drained
3 tablespoons low fat natural yogurt
1 tablespoon lemon juice
1 tablespoon olive oil
salt and pepper
shredded lettuce, to serve (optional)
chopped parsley, to garnish

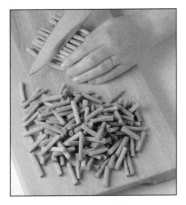

Trim the beans and cut into 2.5 cm (1 in) lengths. Put into a pan of boiling water and cook for 3-4 minutes until just tender.

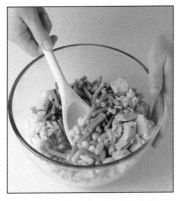

Drain the beans and rinse under cold water to cool. Put the beans into a bowl with the onion, cannellini beans and tuna, and mix together, breaking up the tuna.

Mix the yogurt, lemon juice and oil together, season with salt and pepper and stir into the salad. Serve on a bed of shredded lettuce (if wished) and garnish with chopped parsley.

Serves 4.

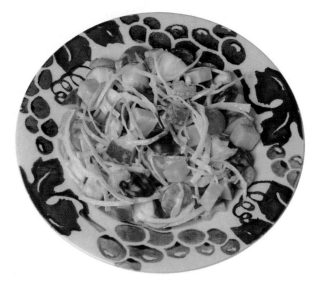

─ FRUITY CHEESE COLESLAW ─

1 red apple
3 teaspoons lemon juice
175 g (6 oz) white cabbage, finely shredded
2 sticks celery, finely sliced
115 g (4 oz) green grapes
115 g (4 oz) black grapes
55 g (2 oz) Cheddar cheese
55 g (2 oz) Gouda cheese
2 tablespoons sunflower oil
2 tablespoons fromage frais or natural yogurt
1 teaspoon clear honey

Core the apple, cut apple into small chunks and toss in the lemon juice.

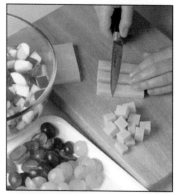

Lift the apple from the juice (reserving juice) and add to the cabbage and celery in a bowl. Cut the grapes in half, remove the pips and add to the salad. Cut the cheeses into small cubes and add to the other ingredients.

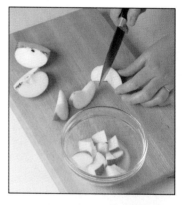

Mix the reserved lemon juice with the oil, fromage frais and honey and whisk until smooth, then fold into the salad.

Serves 4-6.

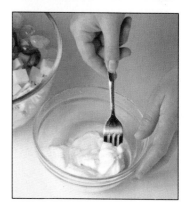

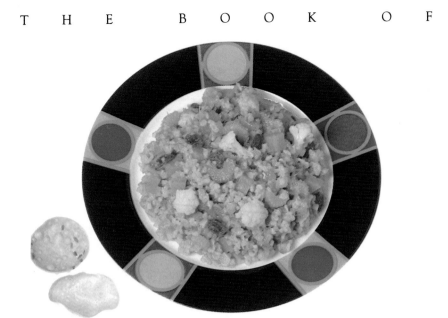

— SPICY VEGETABLE BULGAR —

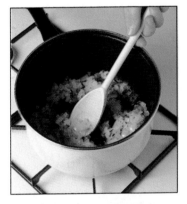

2 tablespoons sunflower oil
1 onion, chopped
175 g (6 oz) bulgar wheat
3 teaspoons mild curry powder
2 carrots, diced
2 sticks celery, chopped
175 g (6 oz) cauliflower flowerets
550 ml (20 fl oz/2½ cups) hot vegetable stock
25 g (1 oz/¼ cup) raisins or sultanas
2 tablespoons fruity chutney
salt and pepper

Heat half the oil in a large saucepan, add the onion and cook until soft, stirring occasionally.

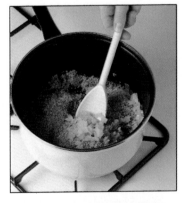

Add the remaining oil, stir in the bulgar wheat and curry powder and cook over a low heat for 1 minute. Add the prepared vegetables, then pour in the stock. Cover and simmer the mixture for 15 minutes.

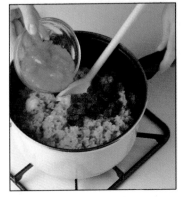

Stir in the raisins or sultanas and the chutney, season to taste and heat through. Serve with small poppadums.

Serves 4-6.

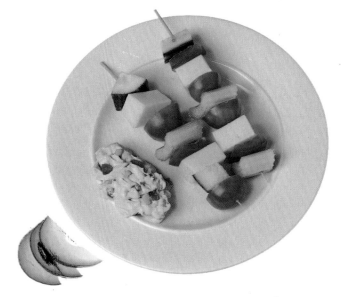

SALAD KEBABS

2 sticks celery, washed
10 cm (4 in) piece cucumber
175 g (6 oz) Gouda or Edam cheese, cubed
1 red pepper (capsicum), seeded and cut into pieces
8 cherry tomatoes, halved
DIP:
2 tablespoons low fat soft cheese
1 ripe avocado
1 tomato, skinned and finely chopped
3 spring onions, finely chopped
salt and pepper

Cut the celery and cucumber into 1-2.5 cm (½-1 in) pieces.

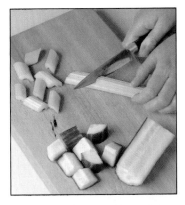

Thread celery and cucumber onto 8 small bamboo skewers with the cheese, pepper (capsicum) and tomato halves.

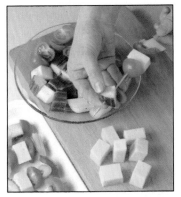

Put the soft cheese into a bowl, halve the avocado, scoop out the flesh, add to the cheese and mash well together. Stir in the chopped tomato and spring onion and season to taste with salt and pepper. Serve as a dip with the kebabs.

Serves 4.

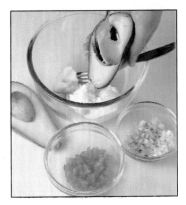

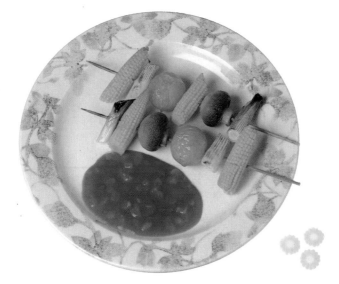

VEGETABLE KEBABS

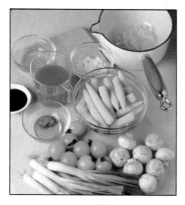

1 bunch thick spring onions, trimmed
470 g (15 oz) can baby sweetcorn, drained
8 cherry tomatoes
115 g (4 oz) button mushrooms, trimmed
oil for brushing
BARBECUE SAUCE:
1 tablespoon oil
1 tablespoon finely chopped onion
2 teaspoons plain flour
150 ml (5 fl oz/⅔ cup) tomato juice
2 teaspoons wine vinegar
2 teaspoons Worcestershire sauce
1 teaspoon clear honey
½ teaspoon mustard powder

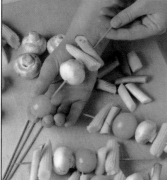

Cut the spring onions into 2.5 cm (1 in) lengths; halve the baby sweetcorn, if large, and arrange with the other vegetables on 8 small bamboo skewers. Brush with oil and place under a hot grill to cook for 5-8 minutes, turning them halfway through the cooking time.

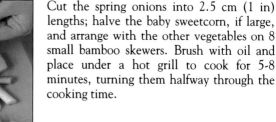

Meanwhile make the sauce. Heat the oil in a small saucepan, add the onion and cook until soft. Stir in the flour, then add the tomato juice and the remaining ingredients and cook for 3 minutes, stirring continuously, until thickened. Serve with the kebabs.

Serves 4.

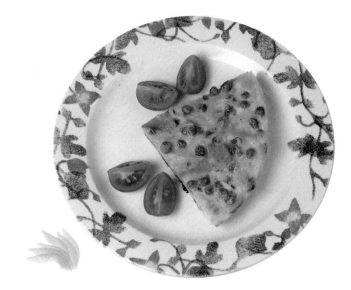

———— SPANISH OMELETTE ————

1 tablespoon olive oil
½ onion, finely chopped
4 bacon rashers, rinded and chopped
½ orange, red or green pepper (capsicum), seeded and
   cut into thin strips
175 g (6 oz) potatoes, grated
4 eggs, beaten
salt and pepper
55 g (2 oz) frozen peas, thawed
2 tomatoes, cut into wedges, to serve

Heat the oil in a medium non-stick frying pan
and cook the chopped onion and bacon until
lightly golden.

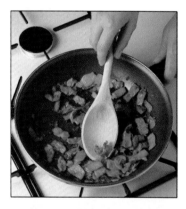

Add the pepper (capsicum) and potato to the
pan and continue to cook for 4-5 minutes
until the potato softens.

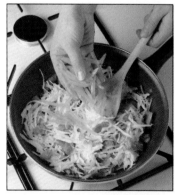

Beat the eggs together with the seasoning and
pour into the frying pan, add the peas and
cook over a medium heat for 5-10 minutes
until the eggs are set. Place the frying pan
under a preheated grill for 1 minute to set the
top of the omelette. Turn out of the pan, cut
into 4 wedges and serve hot, garnished with
wedges of tomato.

Serves 4

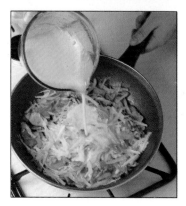

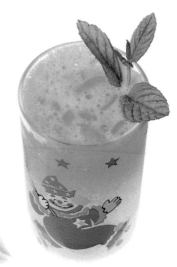

APPLE ZING

2 ripe pears, peeled and cored
450 ml (16 fl oz/2 cups) pure apple juice
crushed ice
550 ml (20 fl oz/2½ cups) chilled ginger ale
apple slices or mint sprigs, to decorate

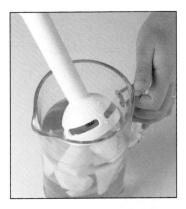

Put the pears and apple juice into a blender and process until smooth, or put them into a jug and blend with a hand blender.

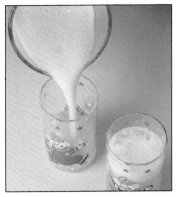

Spoon some crushed ice into 4 tall glasses and pour over the apple juice mixture.

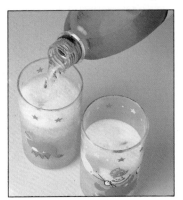

Top up the glasses with the ginger ale and decorate with the apple slices or mint sprigs. Serve immediately.

Serves 4.

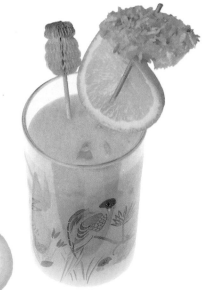

— CARIBBEAN FRUIT COCKTAIL —

6 tablespoons desiccated coconut
200 g (7 oz) can pineapple slices in juice
2 ripe bananas
450 ml (16 fl oz/2 cups) chilled orange juice
crushed ice
1 small orange, sliced

Put 4 tablespoons of the coconut into a pan
with 300 ml (10 fl oz/1¼ cups) water. Bring
to the boil and simmer for 3 minutes, then
allow to cool. Strain the liquid, discarding
the desiccated coconut.

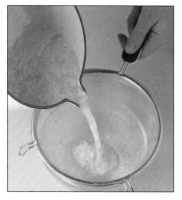

Lightly toast the remaining coconut and set
aside to cool. Reserve 2 pineapple rings for
decoration and put the remainder into a
blender with the pineapple juice, coconut
liquid, peeled bananas and orange juice.
Blend until smooth. Alternatively, put them
into a jug and blend with a hand blender.

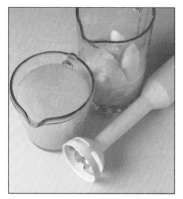

Put crushed ice into 4 glasses and pour the
drink on top. Cut the reserved pineapple
rings into 4-5 pieces and toss in the toasted
coconut. Thread the pineapple pieces onto
wooden skewers or bamboo sticks with the
orange slices and use to decorate each drink.
Serve at once.

Serves 4.

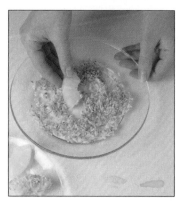

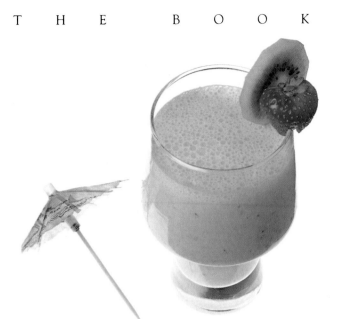

– STRAWBERRY YOGURT WHIZZ –

225 g (8 oz) strawberries
300 ml (10 fl oz/1¼ cups) cold milk
300 ml (10 fl oz/1¼ cups) natural or strawberry yogurt
2 scoops vanilla or yogurt ice cream
1 kiwi fruit (optional)

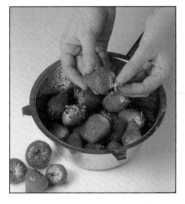

Reserve 4 strawberries for decoration; wash and hull the remainder.

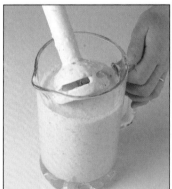

Put the milk, yogurt, strawberries and ice cream into a blender and blend until smooth, or put them into a jug and blend with a hand blender.

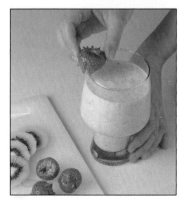

Pour into glasses. Decorate with the reserved strawberries and slices of kiwi fruit, if using.

Serves 3-4.

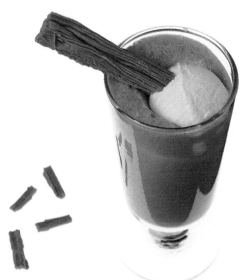

──── MALTED MILKSHAKES ────

410 g (14.5 oz) can evaporated milk
450 ml (16 fl oz/2 cups) chilled milk
3 tablespoons cocoa
2 teaspoons light soft brown sugar
3 tablespoons malt extract
8 scoops vanilla ice cream
4 chocolate flakes

Put 4 glass tumblers in the refrigerator to chill for 30 minutes.

Depending on the size of blender available, either blend in 1 or 2 batches. Put the milks, cocoa, sugar, malt extract and half the ice cream into a jug or blender and blend for 2 minutes until frothy.

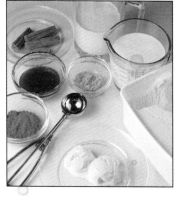

Pour into chilled glasses, top each drink with a scoop of ice cream and a chocolate flake. Serve with straws.

Serves 4.

Variation: Use powdered malted chocolate drink instead of cocoa, if preferred, and reduce the amount of sugar.

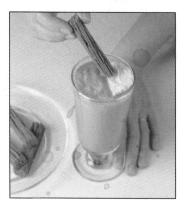

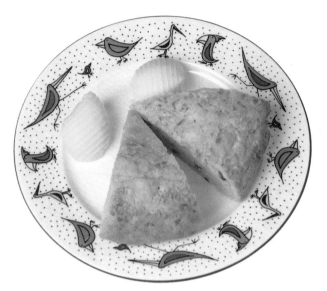

——— SAVOURY SCONES ———

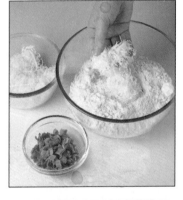

4 bacon rashers, rinded
225 g (8 oz/2 cups) self-raising flour
1 teaspoon baking powder
½ teaspoon salt
1 teaspoon mustard powder
55 g (2 oz/¼ cup) margarine
55 g (2 oz/½ cup) grated Cheddar cheese
8 tablespoons milk, plus extra for brushing

Grill the bacon until crisp, then cut into small pieces. Preheat oven to 220C (425F/Gas 7). Grease a baking sheet.

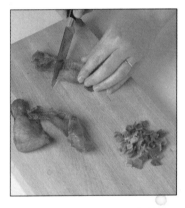

Sift the flour, baking powder, salt and mustard into a bowl. Rub in the margarine, then add three-quarters of the grated cheese and the bacon.

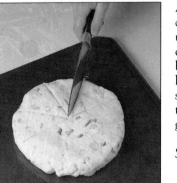

Add the milk and mix to form into a soft dough. Knead on a lightly floured surface until smooth, then press out into a round 15 cm (6 in) in diameter. Place on the greased baking sheet and mark into 8 wedges with a knife. Brush the top with a little milk, then sprinkle with the remaining cheese. Bake in the oven for 12-15 minutes until risen and golden. Cool on a wire rack.

Serves 8.

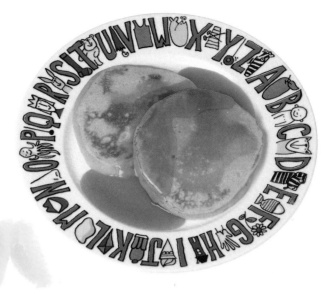

– SAUCY CORNMEAL PANCAKES –

115 g (4 oz/1 cup) plain flour
3 tablespoons caster sugar
1 teaspoon baking powder
150 g (5 oz/1 cup) cornmeal
2 eggs
300 ml (10 fl oz/1¼ cups) milk
2 tablespoons sunflower oil
BUTTERSCOTCH SAUCE:
45 g (1½ oz/9 teaspoons) butter
115 g (4 oz/¾ cup) light soft brown sugar
2 tablespoons golden syrup
3 tablespoons single (light) cream

Put the sauce ingredients in a small pan.

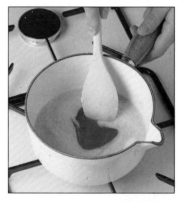

Heat the mixture until the sugar dissolves, stirring all the time. Set aside. In a bowl, put the flour, caster sugar, baking powder and cornmeal. Beat together the eggs, milk and 1 tablespoon of oil, then add to the bowl and beat until the mixture is smooth.

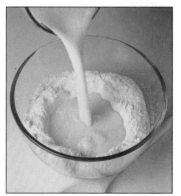

Heat a large, non-stick frying pan over medium-high heat and brush with a little of the remaining oil. Drop 2 or 3 large spoonfuls of the batter into the pan allowing space for them to spread. Cook until bubbles appear on the surface, then turn over and cook the other side until golden. Repeat with the rest of the mixture, keeping the cooked pancakes warm until the rest are cooked. Serve with the butterscotch sauce.

Makes 16.

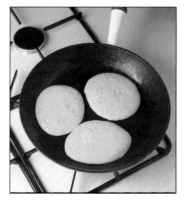

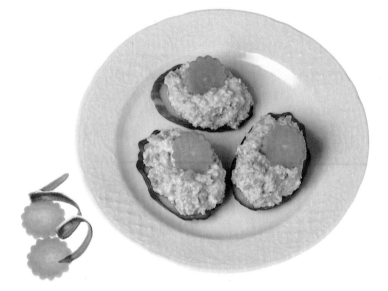

─────CUCUMBER SNACKS─────

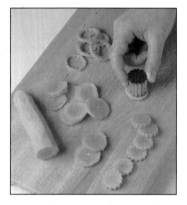

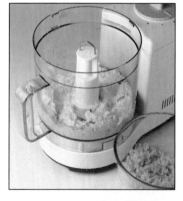

1 large carrot, peeled
2 sticks celery, trimmed
115 g (4 oz/1 cup) sunflower seeds
4 tablespoons natural yogurt
2 tablespoons mayonnaise
1 cucumber

Cut 16 thin slices from the carrot and, using a small fancy cutter, cut out decorations; set aside. Put the trimmings into a food processor with the rest of the carrot and the celery and process until it is finely chopped, then transfer to a bowl.

Put the sunflower seeds, yogurt and mayonnaise into the processor and work until a paste forms. Spoon into the bowl and mix the ingredients together.

Cut 16 slices from the cucumber, cutting on a slant to give diagonal slices. Place a spoonful of the mixture on each and decorate with the carrot shapes.

Makes 16.

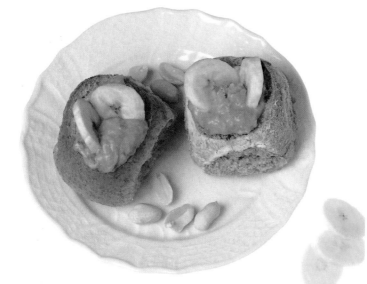

BANANA CUSHIONS

8 mini wholemeal bread rolls
2 tablespoons crunchy peanut butter
2 tablespoons soft cheese
3 small bananas

Cut a small slice off the top of each bread roll. With the point of a sharp knife, scoop out the middle of each one.

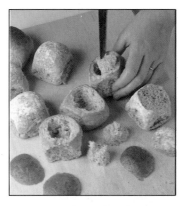

In a bowl, beat together the peanut butter and soft cheese. Roughly mash 2 of the bananas and fold into the mixture. Divide between the bread rolls.

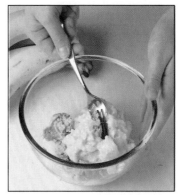

Slice the remaining banana and use to decorate the rolls.

Makes 8.

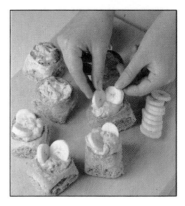

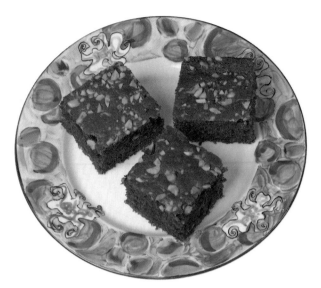

NUTTY BROWNIES

150 g (5 oz/1¼ cups) self-raising wholemeal flour
175 g (6 oz/1 cup) light soft brown sugar
85 g (3 oz/¾ cup) lightly toasted and chopped
 hazelnuts
115 g (4 oz/½ cup) butter
115 g (4 oz) plain (dark) chocolate, broken into small
 pieces
2 eggs, beaten
70 ml (2½ fl oz/⅓ cup) milk
few drops vanilla essence

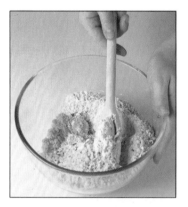

Preheat oven to 180C (350F/Gas 4). Grease a
20 cm (8 in) square shallow baking tin. In a
bowl, mix together the flour, sugar and three-
quarters of the nuts.

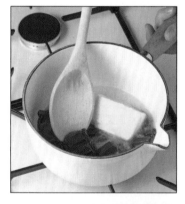

In a saucepan, melt the butter and chocolate
over a low heat. Cool slightly.

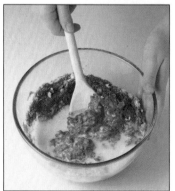

Beat the eggs, milk and vanilla essence
together and add to the flour mixture with
the melted butter and chocolate; beat until
smooth. Pour into the prepared tin, scatter
the remaining nuts over the top and bake in
the oven for 25-30 minutes until firm. Cool
on a wire rack, then cut into 12 pieces.

Makes 12.

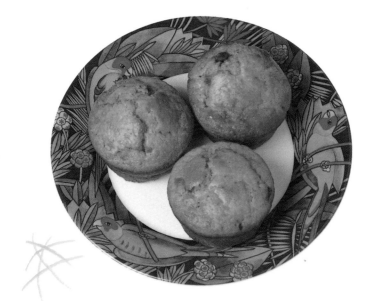

──CHOC & ORANGE MUFFINS──

300 g (10 oz/2 ½ cups) plain flour
3 teaspoons baking powder
pinch salt
85 g (3 oz/½ cup) light soft brown sugar
grated rind and juice 1 orange
2 eggs
250 ml (8 fl oz/1 cup) milk
55 g (2 oz/¼ cup) butter, melted
115 g (4 oz) milk chocolate drops

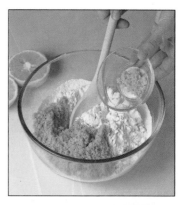

Preheat oven to 200C (400F/Gas 6). Grease 10-12 muffin or deep patty tins or line with paper bun cases. Sift the flour, baking powder and salt into a bowl; stir in the sugar and orange rind.

Beat together the orange juice, eggs, milk and melted butter. Pour onto the dry ingredients, add the chocolate drops and stir together to form a batter. Do not overmix.

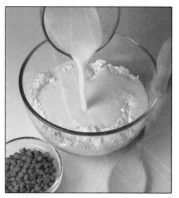

Spoon the mixture into the prepared tins or paper bun cases so they are two-thirds full. Bake in the oven for 20-25 minutes until golden brown and risen.

Makes 10-12.

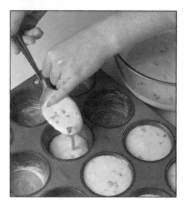

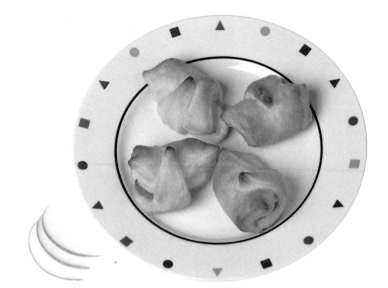

—MINI SAVOURY CROISSANTS—

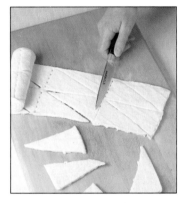

240 g tube of refrigerated ready-to-cook mini
    croissants
115 g (4 oz) Gouda or Cheddar cheese slices
1 small apple
55 g (2 oz) thinly sliced smoked ham
milk, to glaze

Preheat the oven to 200C (400F/Gas 6).
Open the packet of dough as instructed on
the label. Unfold the croissant dough on to a
board and separate the croissants along the
perforations.

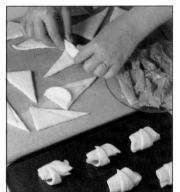

Cut the cheese into small triangles to fit the
croissants and lay a piece on each one. Cut
the apple into 12 small slices and place one at
the broad end on top of the cheese on 12 of
the croissants. Roll each of these croissants
towards the point, then place on a greased
baking sheet.

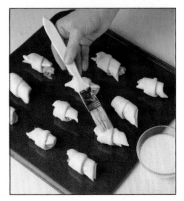

Divide the ham between the remaining 12
croissants and roll up. Place on a baking
sheet. Brush the croissants with milk, then
bake in the oven for 10 minutes until golden
brown. Serve warm.

Makes 24.

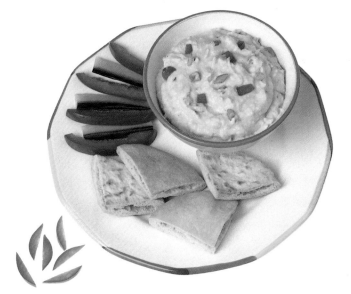

VEGETABLE DIP

400 g (14 oz) can chick peas, drained
1 clove garlic, crushed
4 tablespoons Greek yogurt
½ red pepper (capsicum), seeded and finely diced
3 spring onions, trimmed and finely chopped
salt and pepper
8 small pitta breads

Preheat the oven to 180C (350F/Gas 4). Put the chick peas into a blender or food processor with the garlic and yogurt and work to a purée. Transfer to a bowl.

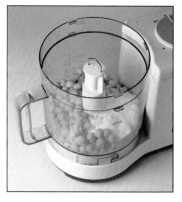

Fold the chopped pepper (capsicum) and the spring onions into the purée and season to taste with salt and pepper.

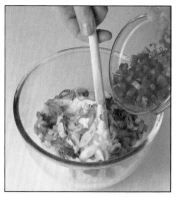

Cut the pitta breads into quarters, place on a baking sheet and put into the oven for about 5 minutes until warm and crisp. Serve at once with the dip.

Serves 4-6.

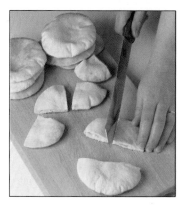

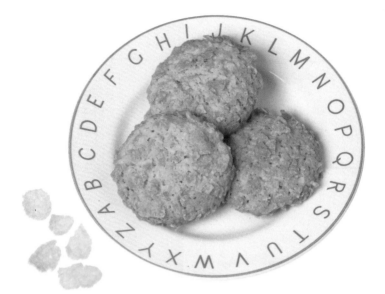

COCONUT CRISPS

150 g (5 oz/²⁄₃ cup) butter or margarine
1 egg
few drops vanilla essence
115 g (4 oz/½ cup) brown sugar
85 g (3 oz/1 cup) desiccated coconut
55 g (2 oz/²⁄₃ cup) rolled oats
115 g (4 oz/1 cup) self-raising flour
55 g (2 oz/2 cups) cornflakes, lightly crushed

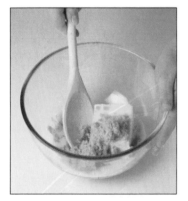

Preheat oven to 170C (325F/Gas 3). Grease 2 baking sheets. Put the butter, egg, vanilla essence and sugar into a bowl and beat together until creamy.

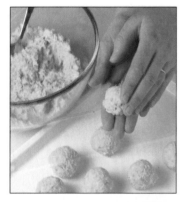

Stir in the coconut, oats and flour and mix to form a dough. Roll the mixture into about 25 balls about the size of a large walnut.

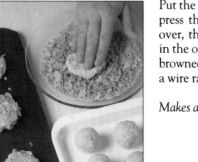

Put the crushed cornflakes on a plate. Lightly press the balls in the cornflakes to coat all over, then place on the baking sheets. Cook in the oven for about 15 minutes until lightly browned. Remove from the oven and cool on a wire rack.

Makes about 25.

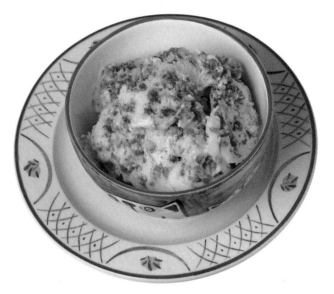

— BROWN BREAD ICE CREAM —

300 ml (10 fl oz/1 ¼ cups) milk
85 g (3 oz/⅓ cup) caster sugar
4 egg yolks
few drops vanilla essence
85 g (3 oz/1 ½ cups) day-old wholemeal breadcrumbs
85 g (3 oz/½ cup) dark soft brown sugar

Heat the milk until just simmering. Beat the caster sugar and egg yolks together in a bowl, then stir in the hot milk. Return to the saucepan and cook over a very low heat until thick, stirring. Allow to cool.

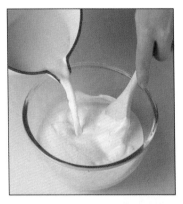

Stir the vanilla essence into the custard, then pour into a shallow dish and freeze until crystals form around the edge of mixture. Remove from the freezer, turn ice cream into a bowl and beat until smooth. Return to the container and freeze again.

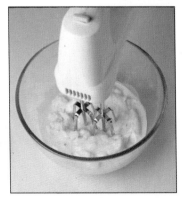

Meanwhile, preheat the oven to 200C (400F/ Gas 6). Mix the breadcrumbs and brown sugar together and spread out on a non-stick baking sheet. Bake in the oven until the crumbs are golden brown, turning during cooking to give an even colour. Allow to cool, then stir into the setting ice cream. Keep frozen until 1 hour before serving, then transfer the ice cream to the refrigerator to soften before serving.

Serve 4-6.

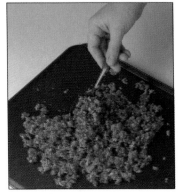

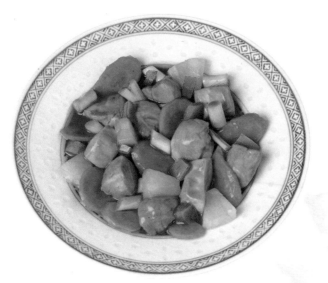

—— SWEET & SOUR CHICKEN ——

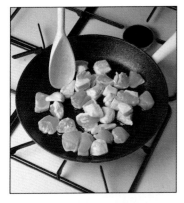

350 g (12 oz) skinless and boneless chicken thighs, cut
   into bite-size pieces
2 tablespoons oil
1 large carrot, thinly sliced
½ green pepper (capsicum), seeded and diced
2 canned pineapple rings, chopped
4 spring onions, chopped
2 tablespoons white wine vinegar
2 tablespoons soy sauce
2 tablespoons tomato ketchup (sauce)
2 tablespoons clear honey
2 teaspoons cornflour
3 tablespoons pineapple juice

Fry the chicken in the oil for 6-8 minutes.

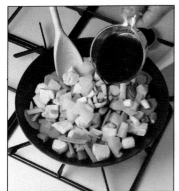

Add the carrot and pepper (capsicum) and
cook for a further 3 minutes. Stir in the
pineapple and spring onions. Mix the
vinegar, soy sauce, tomato ketchup (sauce)
and honey together, then pour into the pan.
Bring to the boil and simmer for 4-5 minutes.

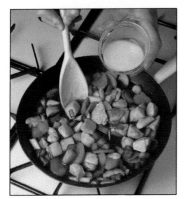

Blend the cornflour with the pineapple juice,
add to the pan and stir until thickened,
stirring all the time. Serve with plain boiled
rice or noodles.

Serve 3-4.

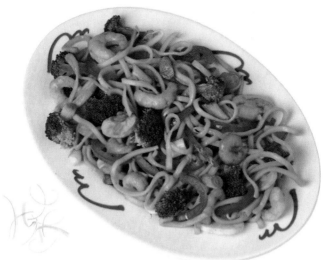

CHOP SUEY SALAD

115 g (4 oz) medium Chinese egg noodles
115 g (4 oz) broccoli flowerets
225 g (8 oz) fresh beansprouts
55 g (2 oz) mushrooms, thinly sliced
5 spring onions, chopped
½ red and ½ green or yellow pepper (capsicum), cut
  into thin slivers
115 g (4 oz) cooked peeled prawns
3 tablespoons sunflower oil
1 tablespoon soy sauce
pinch ground ginger

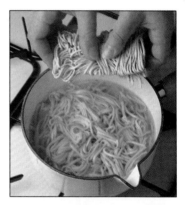

Break the noodles into small pieces and cook in a pan of boiling water for about 3-4 minutes until tender. Drain and cool.

Cut the broccoli into small pieces and blanch in a pan of boiling water for 3 minutes; drain and rinse in cold water, then drain again. Wash the beansprouts and trim the roots, if preferred. Put into a bowl with the mushrooms, onions, peppers (capsicums), prawns, broccoli and noodles.

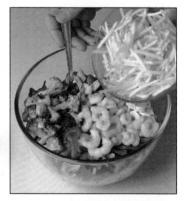

Mix the oil, soy sauce and ginger together. Pour over the salad and toss ingredients lightly together. Serve chilled.

Serves 4.

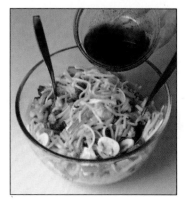

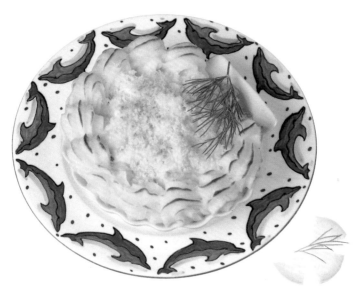

FISHY POTS

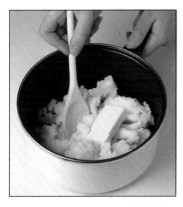

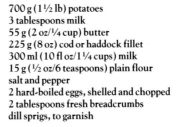

700 g (1½ lb) potatoes
3 tablespoons milk
55 g (2 oz/¼ cup) butter
225 g (8 oz) cod or haddock fillet
300 ml (10 fl oz/1¼ cups) milk
15 g (½ oz/6 teaspoons) plain flour
salt and pepper
2 hard-boiled eggs, shelled and chopped
2 tablespoons fresh breadcrumbs
dill sprigs, to garnish

Cook the potatoes in boiling, salted water until tender. Drain well, return to the pan and mash well. Add the 3 tablespoons milk and half of the butter; beat until smooth.

Put the fish in a pan, add the 300 ml (10 fl oz/ 1¼ cups) milk; cover and poach for 6-7 minutes until the fish flakes easily. Remove the fish and reserve the milk to make a sauce. Flake the fish, discarding skin and bones. Melt the remaining butter in a pan, stir in the flour and cook for 1 minute, then gradually add the milk. Simmer the sauce gently for 1-2 minutes, stirring until thick and smooth, then fold in the fish, seasoning and eggs.

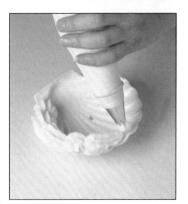

Put the potato into a piping bag fitted with a 1 cm (½ in) star nozzle and pipe a border round the edge of 4 shallow dishes or shells. Spoon the fish mixture into the dishes and scatter over the breadcrumbs. Place under a hot grill until golden. Serve garnished with dill.

Serves 4.

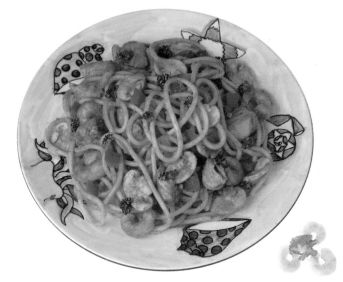

SPAGHETTI MARINARA

225 g (8 oz) spaghetti
1 tablespoon olive oil
1 small onion, finely chopped
1 clove garlic, crushed
115 g (4 oz) button mushrooms, sliced
½ red or green pepper (capsicum), seeded and finely
    diced
300 ml (10 fl oz/1 ¼ cups) passata (sieved tomatoes)
200 g (7 oz) can pink salmon, drained
115 g (4 oz) cooked peeled prawns
pinch dried oregano
salt and pepper

Put the spaghetti into a pan of boiling, salted water and cook until tender; drain.

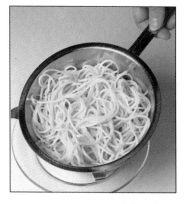

Meanwhile, heat the oil in a saucepan, add the onion, garlic, mushrooms and pepper (capsicum) and cook for 3-4 minutes. Add the passata and simmer for 2-3 minutes. Remove the bones and skin from salmon, then flake and add to the sauce with the prawns. Add the oregano and season to taste.

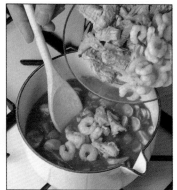

Return the drained spaghetti to the pan, pour over the sauce and toss together to heat through and mix before serving.

Serves 4.

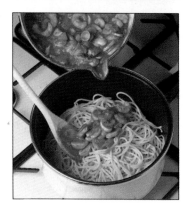

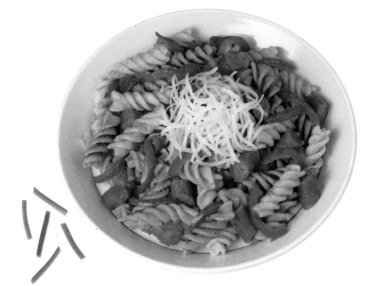

PEPPERAMI PASTA

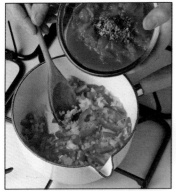

2 tablespoons olive oil
1 onion, finely chopped
1 clove garlic, crushed
1 red pepper (capsicum), seeded and finely sliced
400 g (14 oz) can chopped tomatoes
½ teaspoon sugar
½ teaspoon dried oregano
salt and pepper
225 g (8 oz/4 cups) pasta shapes
115 g (4 oz) pepperami (salami stick), sliced
55 g (2 oz/½ cup) grated Cheddar cheese

Heat the oil in a saucepan, add the onion and cook over a medium heat until softened.

Add the garlic and red pepper (capsicum) and cook briefly. Add tomatoes, sugar and oregano, then season with salt and pepper. Cover and simmer for 10 minutes.

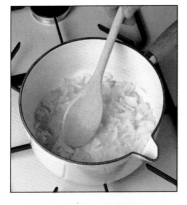

Cook the pasta in a large pan of boiling, salted water for 12 minutes until *al dente* (tender but still with some bite). Drain and return to the pan. Stir in the pepperami and the tomato sauce and heat through. Serve sprinkled with the cheese.

Serves 4.

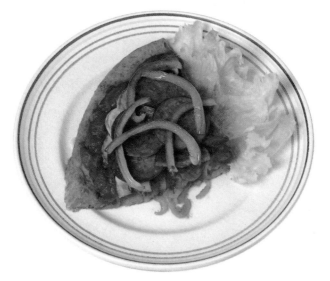

POTATO PIZZA

450 g (1 lb) potatoes, peeled
25 g (1 oz/6 teaspoons) butter
55 g (2 oz/½ cup) plain wholemeal flour
salt
TOPPING:
1 tablespoon olive oil
1 small onion, sliced
200 g (7 oz) can chopped tomatoes
1 tablespoon tomato purée (paste)
½ teaspoon dried basil
55 g (2 oz) button mushrooms, sliced
55 g (2 oz) sliced pizza pepperoni
½ green pepper (capsicum), seeded and cut into thin
    strips

Preheat oven to 200C (400F/Gas 6). Cut the potatoes into even pieces, put into a pan of water and boil until tender. Drain well, mash, then beat in the butter and flour; season with salt. Turn onto a greased baking sheet and spread out to an even round about 20 cm (8 in) in diameter. Bake in the oven for about 10 minutes until the edge of the pizza begins to crisp.

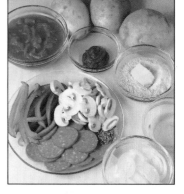

Meanwhile, heat the oil in a small saucepan, add the onion and cook over a medium heat until soft. Stir in the tomatoes, tomato purée (paste) and basil and simmer for 5 minutes until thickened. Spread over the potato base. Arrange the mushrooms over the sauce, then the pepperoni. Place the pepper (capsicum) strips in a criss-cross pattern over the pizza; then bake in the oven for 20 minutes. Serve hot, cut into wedges.

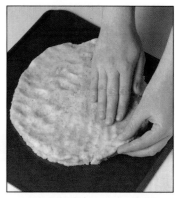

Serve 3-4.

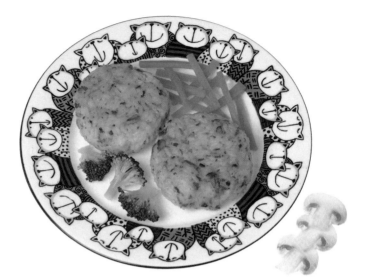

—MUSHROOM & RICE PATTIES—

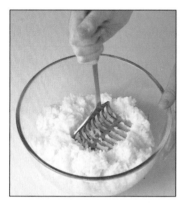

175 g (6 oz/1 ¼ cups) long-grain rice
1 tablespoon sunflower oil
55 g (2 oz) onion, very finely chopped
175 g (6 oz) mushrooms, finely chopped
55 g (2 oz/½ cup) grated Cheddar cheese
salt and pepper
flour
vegetables, to serve

Cook the rice in a pan of boiling, salted water until very tender, Drain well, then put into a bowl and mash to break up the grains. Preheat oven to 200C (400F/Gas 6).

Heat the oil in a medium saucepan, add the onion and mushrooms and cook until all the liquid has evaporated from the mushrooms. Stir into the rice with the cheese and season with salt and pepper.

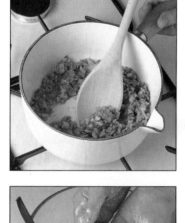

With floured hands, form the mixture into 8 patty shapes and place them on a well greased baking sheet. Bake for 15-20 minutes until golden. Serve with lightly cooked vegetables.

Serves 4.

Variation: Serve with salad and a relish, if preferred.

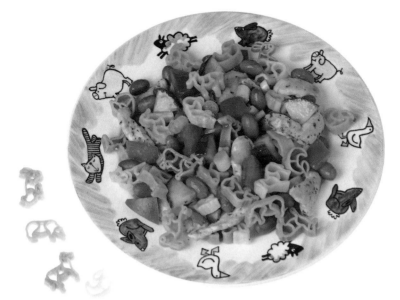

——CHICKEN & PASTA SALAD——

115 g (4 oz) small pasta shapes (such as animals or
 small shells)
350 g (12 oz) boneless chicken breast, skinned
1 teaspoon Italian seasoning
2 tablespoons olive oil
3 tomatoes, seeded and diced
3 spring onions, chopped
5 cm (2 in) piece cucumber, diced
½ x 400 g (14 oz) can borlotti beans
4 teaspoons tomato ketchup (sauce)
2 teaspoons white wine vinegar
chopped parsley, to garnish

Cook the pasta in a pan of boiling, salted
water until tender; drain.

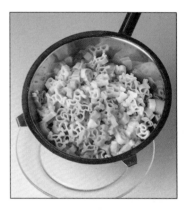

Cut the chicken into small strips and sprinkle
with the Italian seasoning. Heat half the oil
in a non-stick frying pan, add the chicken
and stir over a medium heat about 8-10
minutes until cooked through. Transfer to a
bowl.

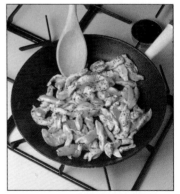

Stir the pasta, tomatoes, onions and cucumber into the bowl with the chicken. Rinse
and drain the beans and add to the salad. Mix
the remaining oil with the tomato ketchup
(sauce) and vinegar, add to the salad and
toss together. Chill until required. Serve
garnished with chopped parsley.

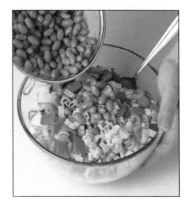

Serves 4.

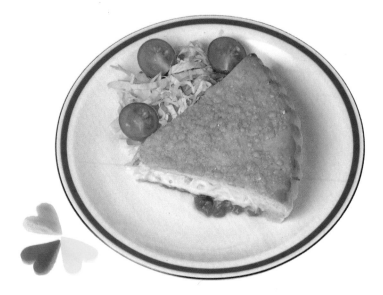

PIZZA PIE

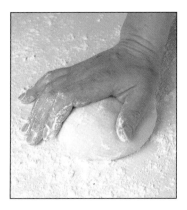

150 g (5 oz) packet pizza dough mix
4 tablespoons tomato pizza topping
85 g (3 oz/¾ cup) grated Mozzarella cheese
85 g (3 oz/¾ cup) grated Cheddar cheese
15 g (½ oz/3 teaspoons) butter
2 tablespoons freshly grated Parmesan cheese

Put the dough mix into a bowl, add 115 ml (4 fl oz/½ cup) warm water and mix to form a dough. Knead for 5 minutes on a lightly floured surface.

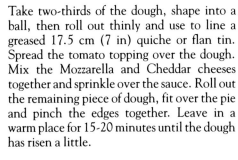

Take two-thirds of the dough, shape into a ball, then roll out thinly and use to line a greased 17.5 cm (7 in) quiche or flan tin. Spread the tomato topping over the dough. Mix the Mozzarella and Cheddar cheeses together and sprinkle over the sauce. Roll out the remaining piece of dough, fit over the pie and pinch the edges together. Leave in a warm place for 15-20 minutes until the dough has risen a little.

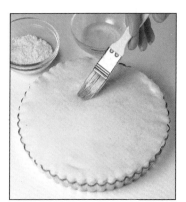

Preheat oven to 200C (400F/Gas 6). Melt the butter, brush over the surface of the pie and scatter the grated Parmesan cheese over the top. Bake in the oven for about 20 minutes until golden and crisp on top.

Serves 3-4.

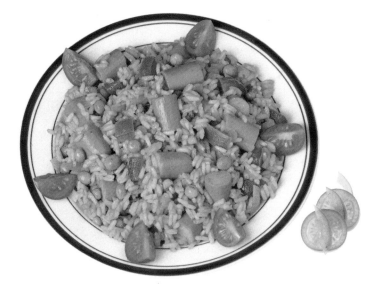

FRANKFURTER RISOTTO

2 tablespoons sunflower oil
1 large onion, chopped
225 g (8 oz/1½ cups) long-grain rice
1 red or green pepper (capsicum), seeded and chopped
450 ml (16 fl oz/2 cups) hot chicken stock
200 g (7 oz) can tomatoes
8 frankfurters
115 g (4 oz) frozen peas
salt and pepper
tomato slices or wedges, to garnish

Heat the oil in a large saucepan, add the onion and cook until the onion softens. Add the rice and pepper (capsicum) and cook for 1 minute, stirring all the time.

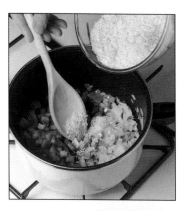

Pour in the stock. Sieve the tomatoes and add the purée to the pan. Bring to the boil, then lower the heat, cover and simmer for 15-20 minutes, or until the rice is tender and all the liquid has been absorbed.

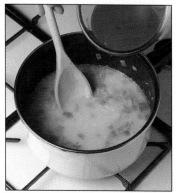

Cut the frankfurters into 1 cm (½ in) long pieces and add to the risotto with the peas; season with salt and pepper. Stir the mixture together over a low heat for about 3 minutes. Garnish with tomato and serve hot.

Serves 4.

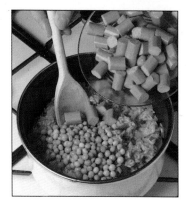

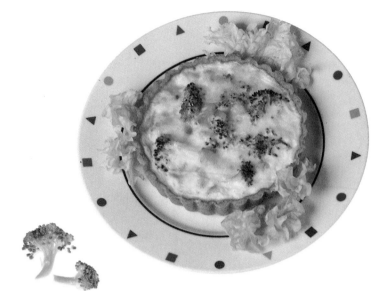

—TURKEY & BROCCOLI FLANS—

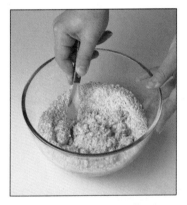

175 g (6 oz/1⅓ cup) plain wholemeal flour
pinch salt
85 g (3 oz/⅓ cup) butter or margarine
2 tablespoons oil
225 g (8 oz) turkey breast meat
175 g (6 oz) broccoli
55 g (2 oz/½ cup) grated Gouda cheese
3 eggs
300 ml (10 fl oz/1¼ cups) milk
salt and pepper

In a bowl, mix together the flour, and salt, then rub in the butter until the mixture resembles breadcrumbs. Mix to a dough with 1 tablespoon oil and 3 tablespoons water.

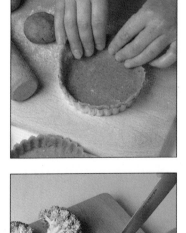

Divide the dough into 6, roll each piece out and use to line six 10 cm (4 in) quiche tins. Place on 2 baking sheets. Preheat oven to 190C (375F/Gas 5). Cut the turkey into small dice. Heat the remaining oil in a non-stick pan and sauté the turkey for 4-5 minutes until white all over. Set aside.

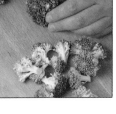

Trim the broccoli into tiny flowerets and blanch in boiling water for 2 minutes; drain well. Divide the cheese between the pastry cases, then add the turkey and broccoli. Beat the eggs and milk together, season and pour into the flans. Bake in the oven for 25-30 minutes until set. Remove from the tins and serve warm or cold.

Makes 6.

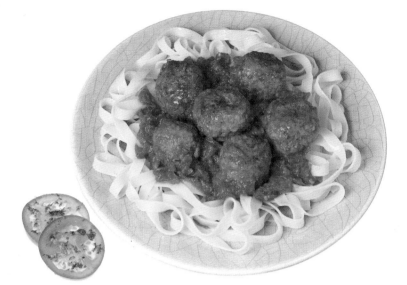

ITALIAN MEATBALLS

1 medium-thick slice wholemeal bread
3 tablespoons milk
450 g (1 lb) lean minced beef
1 clove garlic, crushed
1 tablespoon chopped fresh parsley
1 egg, beaten
salt and pepper
4 tablespoons plain flour
2 tablespoons oil
400 g (14 oz) can tomatoes
1 teaspoon dried oregano
½ teaspoon sugar

Remove crusts from bread. Put bread on a plate, spoon over milk and allow to soak.

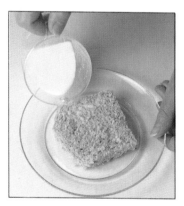

Put the beef, garlic, parsley and egg into a bowl, add the soaked bread, season with salt and pepper and mix until well blended. Divide into 20 small balls, rolling them with wet hands; dust them with the flour.

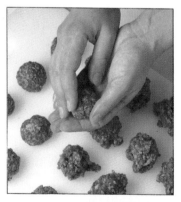

Heat the oil in a large frying pan, add the meatballs and cook until browned all over. Lift out with a slotted and transfer to a large saucepan. Mash the tomatoes, then pour over the meatballs. Add the oregano and sugar and simmer for 20-25 minutes until the tomatoes have thickened to make a sauce. Serve with cooked pasta shapes or tagliatelle.

Serves 4.

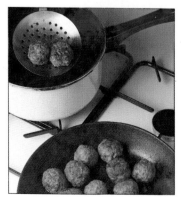

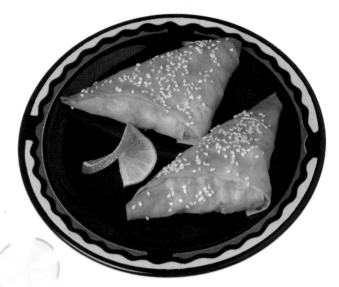

VEGETABLE SAMOSAS

1 tablespoon oil
1 small onion, finely chopped
1 clove garlic, crushed
2 teaspoons mild curry powder
225 g (8 oz) cooked potato, diced
85 g (3 oz) frozen peas
175 g (6 oz) cooked carrots, diced
twelve 32.5 × 23 cm (13 × 9 in) sheets filo pastry
55 g (2 oz/¼ cup) butter, melted
sesame seeds

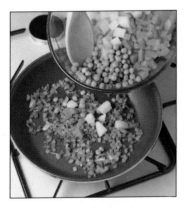

Heat oil in a pan, add onion and garlic; cook until soft. Stir in curry powder and cook for 1 minute. Add potato, peas and carrots and mix together. Allow to cool.

Preheat oven to 190C (375F/Gas 5). Take a sheet of filo pastry and brush lightly with butter. Place a tablespoon of the filling in the middle at the end of strip, then fold the pastry over lengthways. Brush the pastry with melted butter.

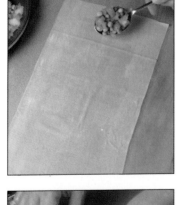

Take the corner of the rectangle and fold it over to make a triangle. Fold the stuffed portion away from you, keeping its three-cornered shape. Continue folding, until you reach the end of the strip. Fill and fold the remaining sheets of pastry in the same way. Place on greased baking sheets, brush with butter and scatter sesame seeds over the top. Bake for about 15 minutes until the samosas are golden and crisp.

Makes 12.

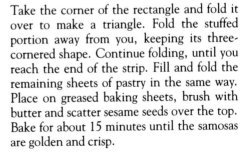

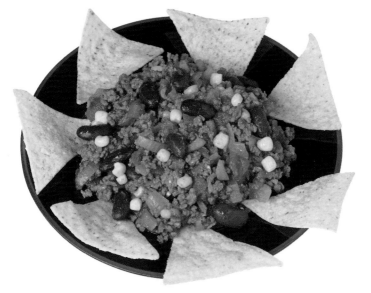

MEXICAN SUPPER

450 g (1 lb) lean minced beef
1 onion, chopped
1 teaspoon mild chilli powder
1 teaspoon ground cumin
400 g (14 oz) can chopped tomatoes
1 tablespoon tomato purée (paste)
200 g (7 oz) can red kidney beans, drained
175 g (6 oz) frozen sweetcorn kernels
salt and pepper
corn chips, to serve

Put the beef, onion and spices into a large, deep frying pan and cook for 4-5 minutes until the meat is browned and the onion is soft, stirring all the time.

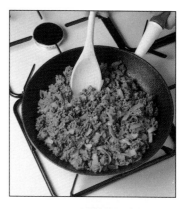

Add the tomatoes and the tomato purée (paste), stir well, then cover and simmer for 15 minutes.

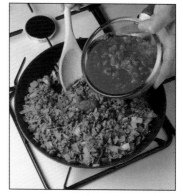

Stir in the red kidney beans and sweetcorn and season with salt and pepper. Continue to cook for 10 minutes. Serve with corn chips.

Serves 4.

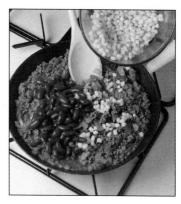

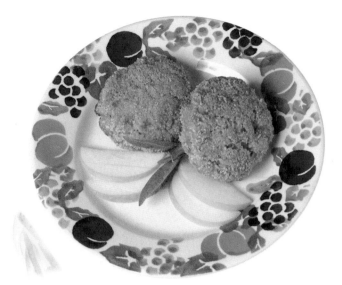

SAUSAGE APPLEBURGERS

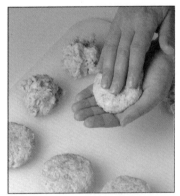

450 g (1 lb) low fat sausagemeat
55 g (2 oz) onion, grated or finely chopped
225 g (8 oz) cooking apple, grated
pinch dried mixed herbs
salt and pepper
2 tablespoons medium oatmeal
apple slices and sage sprigs, to garnish

Preheat oven to 200C (400F/Gas 6). Put the sausagemeat into a large bowl and break up with a fork.

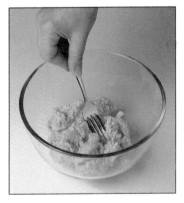

Add the onion, apple and herbs and season with salt and pepper. Mix well until the ingredients are evenly blended, then shape into 8 rounds and flatten them slightly.

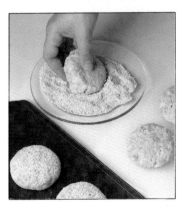

Coat with the oatmeal, then place on a greased baking sheet. Bake in the oven for 25-30 minutes until golden, turning them over halfway through cooking. Serve garnished with slices of apple and sprigs of sage.

Serves 4.

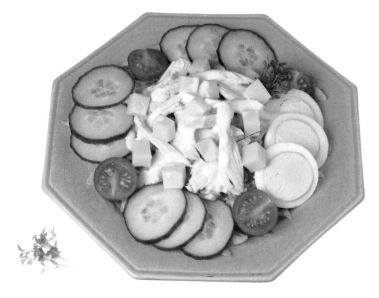

CHEF'S SALAD

½ small iceberg lettuce, shredded
2 carrots, grated
2 eggs, hard-boiled
½ cucumber, sliced
8 cherry tomatoes, halved
175 g (6 oz) cooked chicken, shredded
115 g (4 oz) Edam or Gouda cheese, diced
mustard and cress
DRESSING:
55 ml (2 fl oz/¼ cup) natural yogurt
55 ml (2 fl oz/¼ cup) mayonnaise
2 teaspoons lemon juice
1 tablespoon orange juice

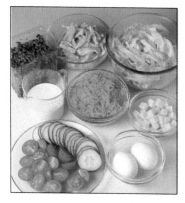

Put the lettuce either into 1 large serving bowl or 4 individual bowls and top with the grated carrot. Slice the eggs and arrange around the side of the bowl (or bowls) with the sliced cucumber and tomatoes. Put the shredded chicken in the middle and scatter over the cheese.

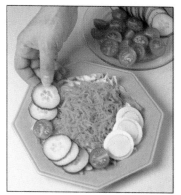

Mix the dressing ingredients together, drizzle it over the salad and then garnish with the mustard and cress.

Serves 4.

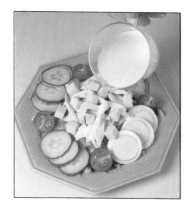

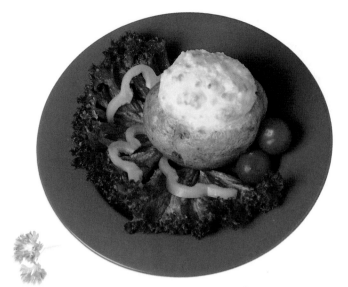

——FLUFFY JACKET POTATOES——

4 potatoes
vegetable oil, for brushing
25 g (1 oz/6 teaspoons) butter
3 eggs, separated
85 g (3 oz/¾ cup) grated Cheddar cheese
salt and pepper
parsley, to garnish

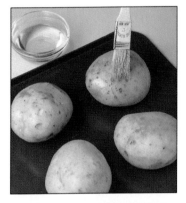

Preheat oven to 200C (400F/Gas 6). Prick the potatoes all over with a fork and brush the skins lightly with oil. Bake in the oven for 45-60 minutes or until the potatoes are cooked.

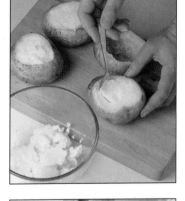

Cut off the tops of the potatoes and scoop out the cooked flesh and put into a bowl, making sure the skin is not pierced. Mash the potato flesh with the butter, then beat in the egg yolks, cheese and seasoning to taste.

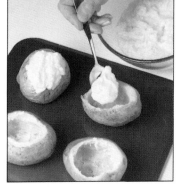

Whisk the egg whites until stiff, then fold into the potato. Spoon back into the potato skins and return to the oven for a further 10-15 minutes. Garnish with parsley.

Serves 4.

Variation: Stir in 55 g (2 oz) chopped cooked ham or 1 tablespoon sweet pickle, if wished.

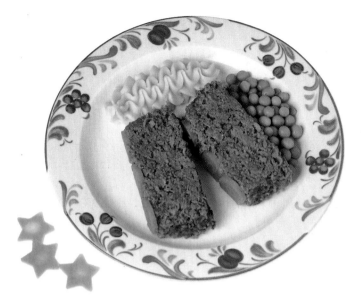

TASTY MEATLOAF

175 g (6 oz) carrots
450 g (1 lb) lean minced beef
55 g (2 oz/1 cup) fresh white or wholemeal
   breadcrumbs
55 g (2 oz) onion, finely chopped
½ teaspoon made mustard
2 tablespoons tomato purée (paste)
1 teaspoon dried mixed herbs
1 egg, beaten
salt and pepper

Preheat oven to 180C (350F/Gas 4). Grease and line a 700 g (1½ lb) loaf tin with grease-proof paper. Thinly slice enough of the carrots to line the base of the tin.

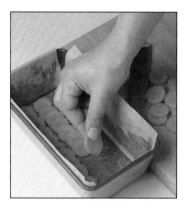

Grate the remaining carrots and put into a bowl with the rest of the ingredients. Mix well and season with salt and pepper.

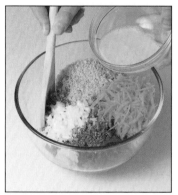

Carefully spoon the mixture into the tin and level the surface. Cover with foil. Bake in the oven for 1 hour until firm. To serve, turn out onto a flat plate and peel off the lining paper. Serve hot or cold.

Serves 4-5.

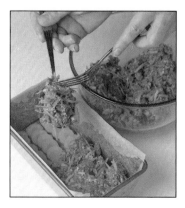

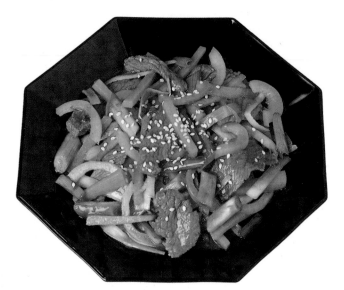

– DANIEL'S FAVOURITE STIR FRY –

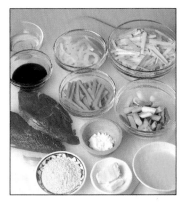

350 g (12 oz) rump steak
2 tablespoons soy sauce
15 g (½ oz) creamed coconut
5 tablespoons boiling water
2 tablespoons sunflower oil
1 clove garlic, crushed
1 large carrot, cut into matchsticks
1 leek, shredded
1 red or yellow pepper (capsicum), seeded and thinly
　sliced
5 spring onions, chopped
2 teaspoons cornflour
3 tablespoons orange juice
sesame seeds
cooked rice or noodles, to serve

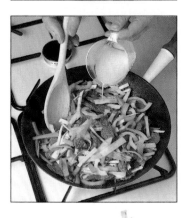

Cut the steak into thin slices, put into a bowl with 1 tablespoon of the soy sauce and mix together. Dissolve the coconut in the boiling water; set aside. Heat the oil in a large frying pan or wok, add the steak and garlic and cook for 3-4 minutes until the steak is almost brown all over.

Add the carrot, leek and pepper (capsicum) and stir fry for a further 3 minutes. Add the coconut mixture, remaining soy sauce and spring onions and bring to simmering point, stirring all the time. Blend the cornflour with the orange juice, add to the pan and cook to thicken the sauce, stirring. Sprinkle over the sesame seeds. Serve at once with rice or noodles.

Serves 4.

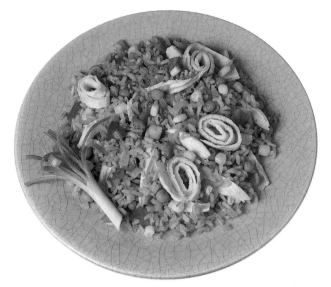

——— CHICKEN FRIED RICE ———

225 g (8 oz/1½ cups) long-grain brown rice
3 tablespoons sunflower oil
1 egg
1 small onion, finely chopped
1 red pepper (capsicum), seeded and chopped
225 g (8 oz) cooked chicken, shredded
55 g (2 oz) frozen peas, thawed
55 g (2 oz) frozen sweetcorn, thawed
3 teaspoons soy sauce
4 spring onions, to garnish

Cook the rice in boiling, salted water for about 20 minutes until just tender. Drain.

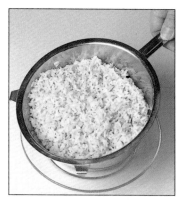

Heat 2 teaspoons oil in a medium frying pan. Beat the egg with 1 tablespoon water, add to the pan and cook until set. Turn onto a board, roll up and cut into thin strips; set aside. Heat the remaining oil in a large frying pan, add the onion and pepper (capsicum) and cook for 2-3 minutes.

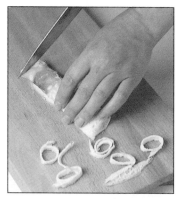

Stir in the rice and fry over a low heat for 3-4 minutes. Add the chicken, peas, sweetcorn and soy sauce and stir fry for 3 minutes. Add the omelette strips to the fried rice and toss together before serving, garnished with spring onions.

Serves 4.

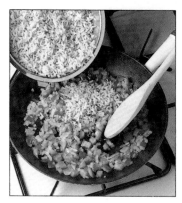

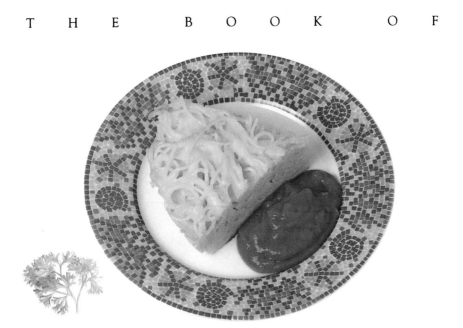

SPAGHETTI FRITTATA

225 g (8 oz) spaghetti
6 teaspoons olive oil
salt
1 onion, finely chopped
4 eggs
115 g (4 oz/1 cup) grated Cheddar cheese
½ clove garlic, crushed
2 teaspoons plain flour
300 ml (10 fl oz/1 ¼ cups) passata (sieved tomatoes)

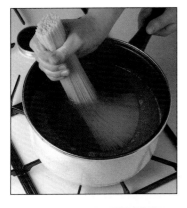

Bring a large pan of water to the boil, add 2 teaspoons oil and 1 teaspoon salt. Add the spaghetti and cook for 8-10 minutes until *al dente* (tender but still with some bite). Drain.

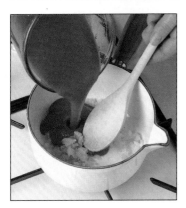

Heat 2 teaspoons oil in a medium frying pan, add half the onion and cook until soft; remove from the heat. In a large bowl, beat the eggs, stir in the cheese and the cooked onion, season with a little salt, then mix in the spaghetti. Turn into the frying pan and set over a medium-low heat to cook for about 10 minutes.

Meanwhile, heat the remaining oil in a small saucepan, add the remaining raw onion and garlic and cook until soft. Stir in the flour, then add the passata, bring to simmering, stirring and cook the sauce for 4-5 minutes. Once the frittata is set, place under a medium-hot grill until lightly golden. Cut into wedges and serve with the sauce.

Serves 4.

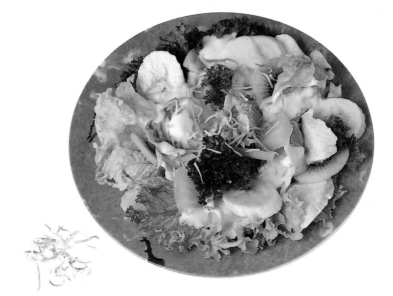

—COCONUT CHICKEN SALAD—

1 lettuce or mixed lettuce leaves
2 portions cooked chicken
2 large bananas
1 kiwi fruit, peeled and sliced
2 canned pineapple rings, cut into pieces
DRESSING:
55 g (2 oz/^{2}/$_3$ cup) desiccated coconut
175 ml (6 fl oz/^{3}/$_4$ cup) boiling water
2 tablespoons mayonnaise
pineapple juice (optional)
toasted coconut, to garnish

First, make the dressing. Put the coconut into a saucepan with the boiling water and then simmer for 2 minutes.

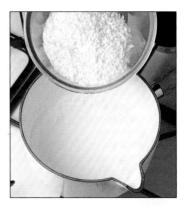

Tip the sauce mixture into a blender or food processor and blend to break down the coconut. Press the pulp through a sieve, pressing with the back of a spoon to extract the liquid. Reserve the coconut pulp.

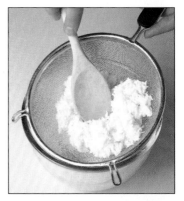

Wash and dry the lettuce leaves and arrange on 4 serving plates, Discard the skin and bones from the chicken and cut into small pieces. Thickly slice the bananas and arrange over the lettuce with the chicken, kiwi fruit and pineapple pieces. Whisk the mayonnaise into the coconut milk, adding a little reserved coconut for a thicker dressing, or a little pineapple juice for a thinner dressing. Spoon over salad; garnish with toasted coconut.

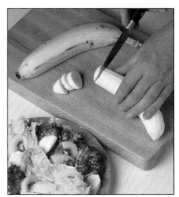

Serves 4.

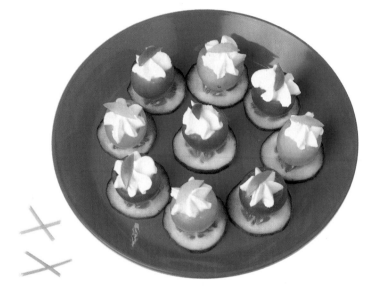

TOMATO FLOWERS

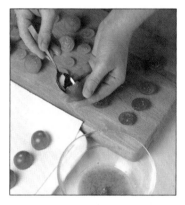

225 g (8 oz) cherry tomatoes, use yellow ones if
  available
175 g (6 oz/³⁄₄ cup) medium fat soft cheese
¹⁄₂ cucumber, sliced
chives, to garnish

Cut the tops off the tomatoes and reserve.
Scoop out the tomato centres, then place
upside-down on a double thickness of absorbent kitchen paper to drain.

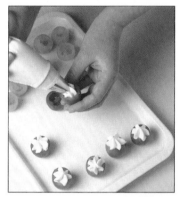

Beat the cheese to soften and place in a
piping bag fitted with a small star nozzle. Pipe
the cheese into the tomatoes.

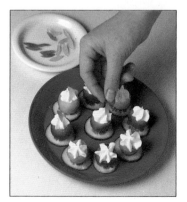

Arrange slices of cucumber on a serving plate
and place the tomatoes on top. Cut tiny
pieces of tomato from the reserved tops and
use to decorate the tomatoes. Garnish with
strands of chives.

Serves 6-8.

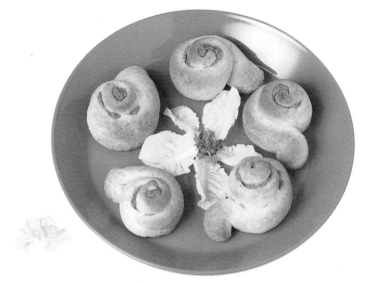

PEANUT SNAILS

175 g (6 oz/1½ cups) self-raising flour
½ teaspoon mustard powder
85 g (3 oz/⅓ cup) sunflower margarine
55 g (2 oz/½ cup) grated Cheddar cheese
3 tablespoons milk
peanut butter
salad, to serve

Preheat the oven to 190C (375F/Gas 5). Sift the flour and mustard powder into a bowl, then rub in the margarine until the mixture resembles fine breadcrumbs. Stir in the cheese, then bind together with the milk to make a fairly soft dough.

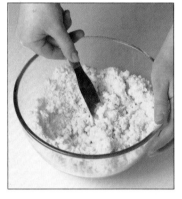

Turn the dough onto a floured surface and knead lightly until smooth. Roll into a sausage shape about 30 cm (12 in) long. Cut into 20 slices. Take each slice and roll out into a thin sausage shape about 15 cm (6 in) long. Gently press three-quarters of the length to make this part of the dough about 1 cm (½ in) wide.

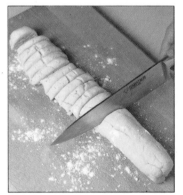

Spread a little peanut butter along the flattened surface, then roll up towards the unflattened end to make a snail shape. Form a head at the end and transfer to a greased baking sheet. Repeat the process with the other pieces of dough. Bake in the oven for 12-15 minutes until golden. Cool on a wire rack. Serve with salad.

Makes 20.

Variation: Yeast extract can be used instead of peanut butter, if wished.

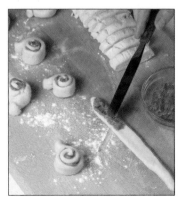

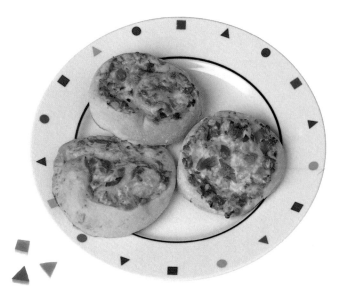

—————— PIZZA SWIRLS ——————

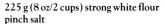

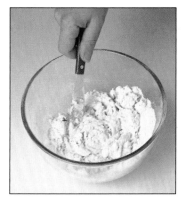

225 g (8 oz/2 cups) strong white flour
pinch salt
1 sachet easy blend dried yeast
200 ml (7 fl oz/1 cup) warm water
150 ml (5 fl oz/²⁄₃ cup) passata (sieved tomatoes)
2 tablespoons tomato purée (paste)
1 clove garlic, crushed
1 teaspoon dried oregano
200 g (7 oz) can tuna, drained and mashed
1 red or green pepper (capsicum), seeded and chopped
1 small onion, finely chopped
85 g (3 oz/²⁄₃ cup) grated Mozzarella cheese

Sift the flour and salt into a bowl, add the yeast and warm water. Mix to a soft dough.

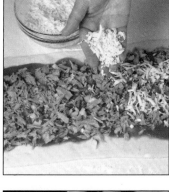

Turn the dough onto a lightly floured work surface and knead for 10 minutes. Roll out to a rectangle about 40 × 20 cm (16 × 8 in). Mix the passata, tomato purée (paste), garlic and oregano together and spread over the dough. Mix the tuna with the pepper (capsicum) and onion and spoon over the dough; scatter the cheese over the top.

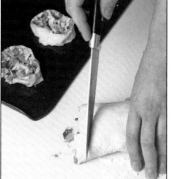

Roll up from a long side, then cut into 1 cm (½ in) slices). Place slices, cut side up, on greased baking sheets and leave in a warm place for 15 minutes. Meanwhile, preheat oven to 190C (375F/Gas 5). Bake the pizza swirls for 15 minutes until golden brown. Serve warm.

Makes about 25-30.

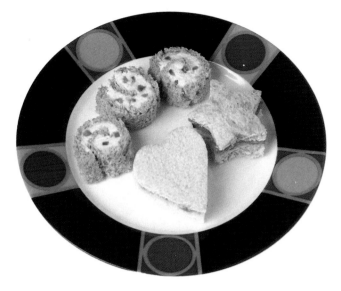

——— PARTY SANDWICHES ———

PINWHEELS:
4 slices wholemeal bread
sunflower margarine or butter, for spreading
115 g (4 oz/½ cup) soft cream cheese
85 g (3 oz/¾ cup) grated Cheddar cheese
2 tablespoons finely chopped red pepper (capsicum)
HEARTS:
6 slices white or wholemeal bread
99 g (3½ oz) can tuna, drained
2 tablespoons low fat soft cheese
STARS:
6 slices mixed grain bread
12 small slices salami, ham or garlic sausage
cucumber slices

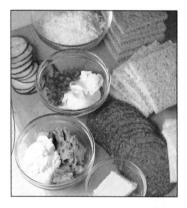

To make the pinwheel sandwiches, remove the crusts from the bread and roll the slices to flatten slightly. Spread bread with a little margarine. Make the filling by mixing together the cheeses and pepper (capsicum). Spread over the bread, then roll up each slice like a Swiss roll. To make the heart-shaped sandwiches, cut out heart shapes from the slices of bread and spread a little margarine on one side. Mash the tuna and low fat cheese together until soft and use to fill the small heart-shaped sandwiches.

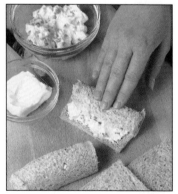

To make the star-shaped sandwiches, cut out stars from the bread, salami and cucumber. Lightly spread the bread with margarine and make up each star with a piece of salami and cucumber. Cover and chill all the sandwiches until needed. To serve the pinwheels, unwrap and cut each into 4 slices. Serve with the stars and hearts.

Makes 40 assorted sandwiches.

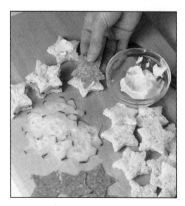

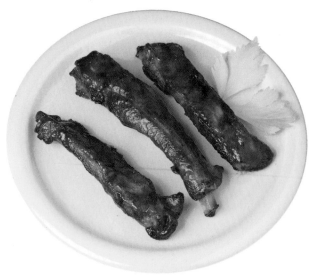

STICKY RIBS

700 g (1½ lb) pork spare ribs (sheets)
5 tablespoons tomato ketchup (sauce)
2 tablespoons clear honey
1 tablespoon soy sauce
1 tablespoon wine vinegar
1 tablespoon Worcestershire sauce
2 tablespoons orange juice

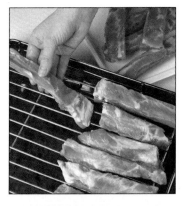

Preheat oven to 200C (400F/Gas 6). Cut the ribs into single rib pieces, if necessary. Arrange on a roasting rack set over a roasting tin. Pour a little water into the tin and bake in the oven for 25 minutes.

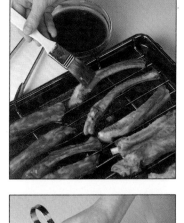

Meanwhile, mix the remaining ingredients together. Brush the ribs on both sides with the glaze. Reduce the oven temperature to 180C (350F/Gas 4) and continue cooking ribs for a further 15 minutes.

Turn the ribs over, brush again with the glaze and cook for a further 15-20 minutes until richly golden. Serve hot with salad.

Serves 6.

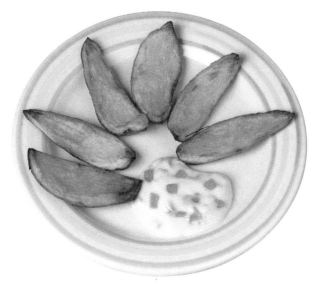

——————PARTY POTATO SKINS——————

1 kg (2.2 lb) potatoes
3 tablespoon olive oil
salt
CHEESE AND HAM SAUCE:
15 g (½ oz/3 teaspoons) butter
25 g (1 oz/¼ cup) plain flour
300 ml (10 fl oz/1¼ cups) milk
55 g (2 oz/ ½ cup) grated Cheddar cheese
55 g (2 oz) ham, finely diced
pinch cayenne pepper (optional)

Cut the unpeeled potatoes lengthways into even, wedge-shaped pieces. Cook in boiling water for 5 minutes, then drain.

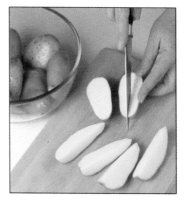

Preheat oven to 220C (425F/Gas 7). Leave the potato wedges until cool enough to handle, then cut out the flesh leaving about 0.5 cm (¼ in) potato attached to the skin. Place the skins on a baking sheet and brush with the oil, then sprinkle with salt and bake in the oven for about 20 minutes until crisp.

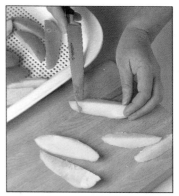

Meanwhile, make the sauce. Melt the butter in a small saucepan, stir in the flour, then gradually add the milk. Cook, stirring all the time until thickened. Stir in the cheese and ham, reheat gently and season with cayenne pepper, if wished. Serve warm with the potato skins.

Serve 6-8.

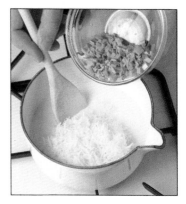

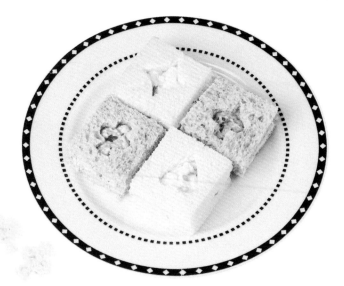

—PLAYING CARD SANDWICHES—

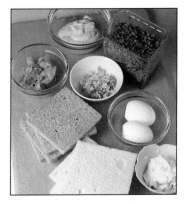

4 slices wholemeal bread, crusts removed
4 slices white bread, crusts removed
sunflower margarine
SALMON FILLING:
1 tablespoon mayonnaise
2 teaspoons lemon juice
99 g (3½ oz) can red salmon
½ carton mustard and cress
EGG FILLING:
2 eggs, hard-boiled
1 tablespoon mayonnaise
2 spring onions, finely chopped

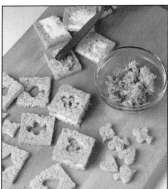

Cut each slice of bread into 4. Using half the squares, cut out playing card symbols from the centre of each one. Make the salmon filling. In a small bowl, beat the mayonnaise and lemon juice together. Discard the bones and skin from the salmon, add to the bowl and mash together; stir in the trimmed cress. Lightly spread margarine over the 8 whole squares of wholemeal bread. Spread over the salmon filling, then cover with the cut out wholemeal squares.

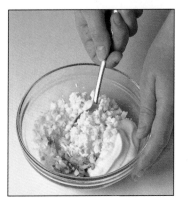

Make the egg filling. In a small bowl, mash the eggs finely; stir in the mayonnaise and onion. Make up the egg sandwiches in the same way as for the salmon sandwiches using the white bread.

Makes 16 sandwiches.

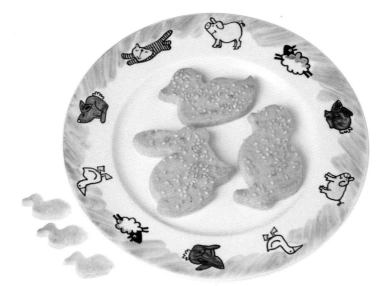

──ANIMAL CHEESE BISCUITS──

115 g (4 oz/1 cup) plain flour
½ teaspoon dry mustard
55 g (2 oz/¼ cup) butter or block margarine
55 g (2 oz/½ cup) grated mature Cheddar cheese
1 egg, beaten
sesame seeds

Preheat oven to 180C (350F/Gas 4). Grease 2 baking sheets. Sift the flour and mustard into a bowl, then rub in the butter until the mixture resembles breadcrumbs.

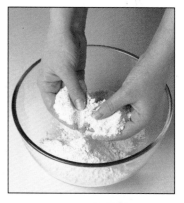

Stir in the cheese, then add 2 tablespoons beaten egg and mix together to make a smooth dough. Turn onto a floured surface, knead lightly, then roll out to about 0.5 cm (¼ in) thickness.

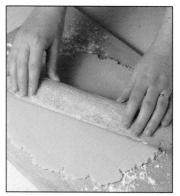

Using animal-shaped cutters, cut out biscuits and place them on the baking sheets. Brush the tops with the remaining egg and sprinkle with sesame seeds. Bake in the oven for 12-15 minutes until golden. Cool on a wire rack.

Makes about 18.

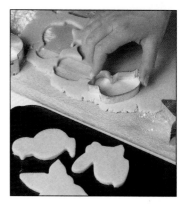

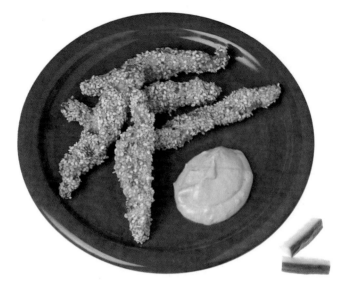

—SESAME CHICKEN FINGERS—

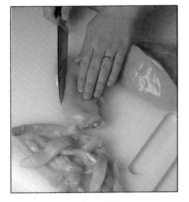

700 g (1½ lb) skinless chicken breast
3 tablespoons plain flour
2 teaspoons tandoori spice mix
salt and pepper
2 eggs
225 g (8 oz/1½ cups) sesame seeds
SAUCE:
4 tablespoons mayonnaise
2 teaspoons tomato purée (paste)
2 tomatoes, skinned, seeded and chopped
1 small clove garlic, crushed

Preheat oven to 200C (400F/Gas 6). Cut the chicken into strips about 1 cm (½ in) wide.

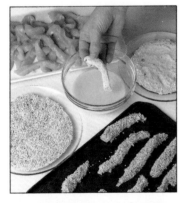

Mix the flour and tandoori spice mix together and season with salt and pepper. Beat the eggs and pour into a shallow dish. Dust the chicken strips with the flour mixture, then dip into the beaten egg. Toss in the sesame seeds and transfer to a greased baking sheet. Bake in the oven for 20-25 minutes.

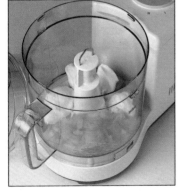

Meanwhile, put all the ingredients for the sauce into a blender or food processor and blend until smooth. Serve with the cooked chicken strips.

Serves 6-8.

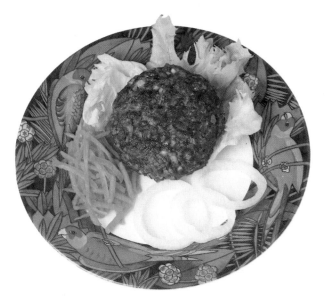

——SURPRISE BEEFBURGERS——

575 g (1¼ lb) lean minced beef
1 small onion, finely chopped
1 teaspoon dried mixed herbs
55 g (2 oz/⅔ cup) rolled oats
1 egg, beaten
salt and pepper
85 g (3 oz) piece cheese (such as Gouda)
1 tablespoon oil
lettuce and grated carrot salad and onion rings, to serve

Put the beef, onion, herbs and oats into a bowl and mix together to break up the beef. Add the beaten egg and seasoning to taste and bind together.

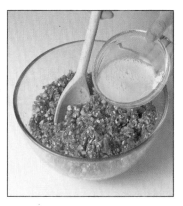

With floured hands, divide the mixture into 6, then flatten each each piece on a board or work surface. Cut the cheese into 6 and place a piece in the middle of each round of meat.

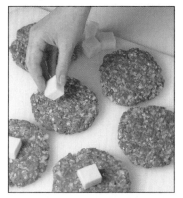

Carefully enclose the cheese in the meat mixture and form into a burger shape. Brush with oil, place under a medium hot grill and cook for about 4-5 minutes on each side until golden. Serve with lettuce and carrot salad and onion rings.

Serves 6.

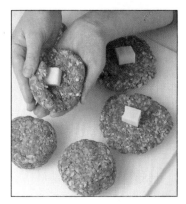

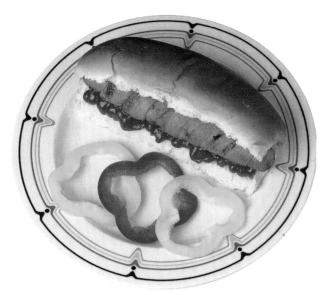

─── SAUSAGE TWISTS ───

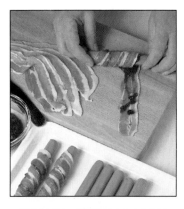

8 rashers streaky bacon, rind removed
2-3 tablespoons barbecue relish
8 frankfurters
8 long bread rolls
tomato ketchup (sauce) or extra barbecue relish,
    to serve

Spread each bacon rasher with relish and wrap around each frankfurter.

Secure each end of the bacon with a cocktail stick. Arrange on a grill rack and place it as far away from the heat as possible.

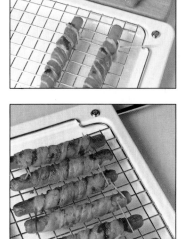

Cook the sausage twists until the bacon is crisp and just lightly browned, turning frequently during cooking. Serve in split, long bread rolls with extra tomato ketchup (sauce) or barbecue relish.

Makes 8.

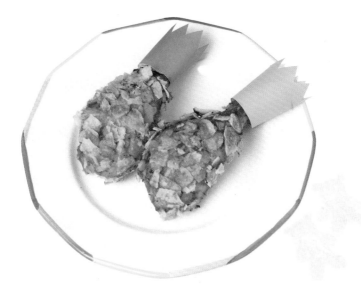

— SPICY CHICKEN DRUMSTICKS —

8 chicken drumsticks
2 tablespoons tomato ketchup (sauce)
1 tablespoon clear honey
3 teaspoons barbecue spice
two 30 g packets plain crisps

Preheat oven to 190C (375F/Gas 5). Using a sharp knife, remove the skin from the chicken legs.

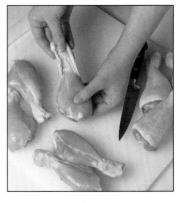

Mix the ketchup (sauce), honey and barbecue spice together and brush over the drumsticks until coated.

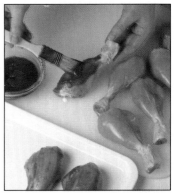

Lightly crush the crisps and roll the drumsticks in them to coat. Place on a rack in a roasting tin and bake for 30 minutes until golden. Pierce a leg with a skewer to check the juices run clear; if they are still pink, cook a little longer before testing again.

Makes 8.

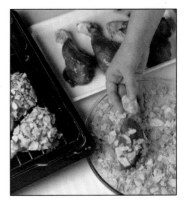

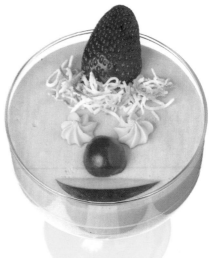

CLOWN TRIFLES

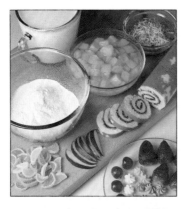

1 small jam Swiss roll
400 g (14 oz) can fruit cocktail
two 69 g (2.4 oz) packets instant whip dessert
  (butterscotch, peach or strawberry flavour)
550 ml (20 fl oz/2½ cups) milk
TO DECORATE:
6 tablespoons long strands of dried coconut, lightly
  toasted
3 large strawberries, halved
12 sugar stars
6 glacé cherries
6 slices red apple
orange and lemon slices

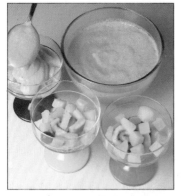

Slice the Swiss roll and place a slice in the bottom of 6 small dishes or teacups. Drain the fruit and spoon over the cake. Make up the dessert whip with the milk as instructed on the packet, then spoon into the dishes, dividing it equally between them.

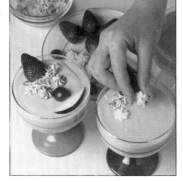

When set, decorate each trifle to look like a clown. Arrange coconut to look like 'hair'; a strawberry half for a hat; sugar stars for 'eyes'; a glacé cherry for the 'nose' and an apple slice for the 'mouth'. Place on a plate and arrange orange and lemon slices around the dish to look like a ruffle.

Serves 6.

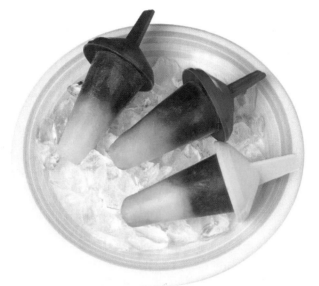

——————— RAINBOW LOLLIES ———————

115 ml (4 fl oz/½ cup) orange juice
85 g (3 oz) fresh raspberries or strawberries
1 teaspoon caster sugar
8 tablespoons blackcurrant cordial

Pour the orange juice into the compartments of a plastic lolly maker. Place in the freezer and leave until hard.

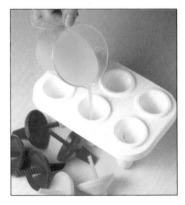

Put the raspberries or strawberries into a blender with the sugar and 4 tablespoons cold water and blend to form a purée. Pass the mixture through a sieve, then pour over the frozen orange layer. Return to the freezer for about 1 hour until almost frozen.

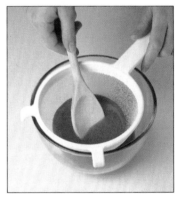

Mix the blackcurrant cordial with 4 tablespoons water, then pour over the raspberry layer. Insert the holders and put into the freezer and leave until solid. To unmould, dip the lolly maker in a bowl of hot water for a few seconds and turn the rainbow lollies out. Serve at once.

Makes about 4, depending on size of lolly maker.

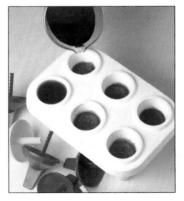

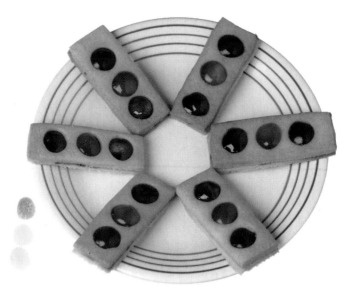

──TRAFFIC LIGHT BISCUITS──

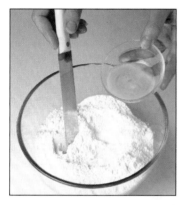

225 g (8 oz/2 cups) plain flour
85 g (3 oz/½ cup) icing sugar
150 g (5 oz/⅔ cup) butter
1 egg yolk
4 tablespoons strawberry jam
2 tablespoons apricot jam
2 tablespoons lime marmalade

Sift the flour and icing sugar into a bowl, then rub in butter until the mixture resembles breadcrumbs. Add the egg yolk and mix to form a dough. Turn onto a floured surface and knead until smooth. Wrap and chill for at least 30 minutes.

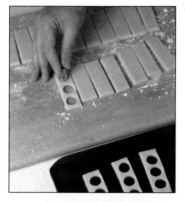

Preheat the oven to 170C (325F/Gas 3). Halve the dough, roll out one half to a 25 × 15 cm (10 × 6 in) oblong. Cut in half lengthways, then cut each half crossways into ten 2.5 cm (1 in) strips. Place on a greased baking sheet. Repeat the procedure with the other half of the dough and cut out 3 circles from each of the strips; discard the circles. Transfer the remaining part of these strips to a greased baking sheet. Bake in the oven for 12 minutes until lightly golden. Leave to cool on the baking sheet.

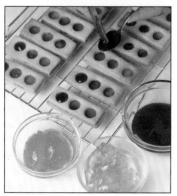

Using half the strawberry jam, spread a thin layer over the plain biscuits. Place the biscuits with holes in on top of them. Sieve the rest of the strawberry jam and fill one hole of each biscuit. Repeat with the apricot jam and the lime marmalade to represent traffic lights.

Makes 20.

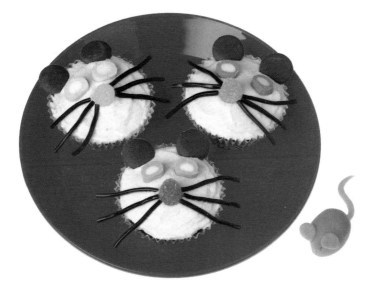

MERRY MICE CAKES

115 g (4 oz/1 cup) self-raising flour
25 g (1 oz/¼ cup) cocoa
115 g (4 oz/½ cup) sunflower margarine
115 g (4 oz/¾ cup) light soft brown sugar
2 eggs, beaten
2 tablespoons milk
DECORATIONS:
175 g (6 oz/1 cup) icing sugar
85 g (3 oz/⅓ cup) butter, softened
chocolate buttons
jelly sweets
liquorice strands and sweets

Put all the ingredients for the cakes into a bowl and beat until smooth.

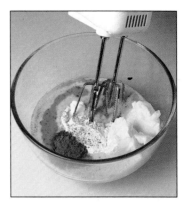

Preheat oven to 180C (350F/Gas 4). Divide the cake mixture evenly between 20 paper bun cases placed in a tartlet tin. Bake the cakes in the oven for about 15 minutes until risen and firm to the touch. Cool on a wire rack. Trim the tops if they have peaks.

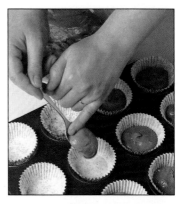

To decorate, beat the icing sugar and butter together until light and fluffy. Spread over the tops of the cakes. Attach 2 chocolate buttons on each cake for 'ears', and place a jelly sweet in position for the 'nose'. Cut slices of liquorice sweets to make 'eyes'. Cut lengths of liquorice strand to make 'whiskers' and insert three on each side of the 'nose'.

Makes 20.

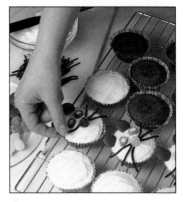

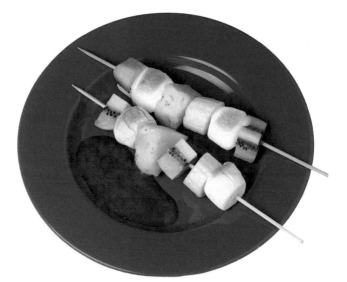

MARSHMALLOW FRUIT KEBABS

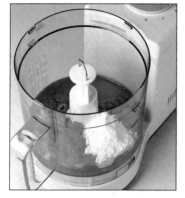

2 firm bananas
2 thick slices pineapple, trimmed
2 kiwi fruit, cut into 2 cm (¾ in) pieces
24 marshmallows
1 tablespoon honey
1 tablespoon lemon juice
RASPBERRY SAUCE:
225 g (8 oz) raspberries, fresh or frozen, thawed if
    frozen
juice 1 orange
1 tablespoon icing sugar

Make the sauce. Put all the sauce ingredients
in a food processor or blender and blend until
smooth. Press through a sieve.

Cut the bananas into thick slices and the
pineapple into chunks. Thread all the fruit
onto 12 oiled bamboo skewers with the
marshmallows. Mix the honey and lemon
juice together and brush over the fruit.

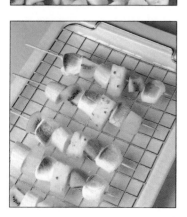

Cook the kebabs under a medium hot grill
until the marshmallows begin to colour, turning once during cooking. Serve with the
raspberry sauce.

Makes 12.

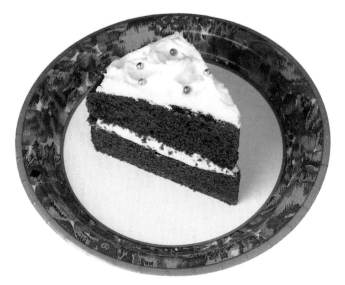

DEVIL'S FOOD CAKE

225 g (8 oz/2 cups) self-raising flour
55 g (2 oz/½ cup) cocoa
150 g (5 oz/⅔ cup) butter
225 g (8 oz/1 ½ cups) dark soft brown sugar
3 eggs, beaten
150 ml (5 fl oz/⅔ cup) milk
few drops vanilla essence
FROSTING:
1 egg white
175 g (6 oz/¾ cup) caster sugar
¼ teaspoon cream of tartar
few drops vanilla essence

Preheat the oven to 180C (350F/Gas 4). Sift the flour with the cocoa.

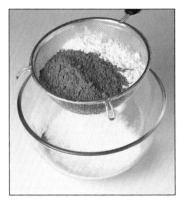

Cream the butter and sugar together, beat in the eggs a little at a time. Fold in the flour mixture until smooth, then add the milk and vanilla essence. Grease and line a 20 cm (8 in) deep cake tin. Spoon the cake mixture into the tin and bake in the oven for about 40 minutes. Cool for 10 minutes before turning out onto a wire rack. Peel away lining paper.

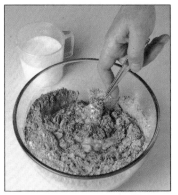

Put all the frosting ingredients into a bowl with 2 tablespoons cold water; stand over a pan of simmering water. Whisk for about 10 minutes until smooth, white and standing in peaks. Cut the cake in half, level the top. Sandwich together with half the frosting and cover with remaining frosting. Leave for 1 hour for the frosting to form a crust.

Serves 8-10.

Variation: Decorate with edible sugar balls or sweets, if wished.

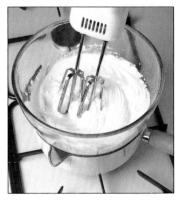

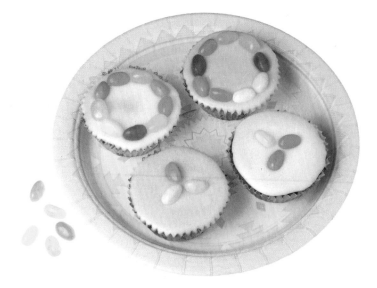

ICED CUP CAKES

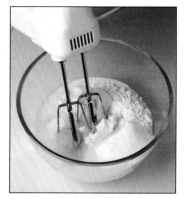

150 g (5 oz/1¼ cups) self-raising flour
115 g (4 oz/½ cup) caster sugar
115 g (4 oz/½ cup) sunflower margarine
2 eggs
2 tablespoons milk
few drops vanilla essence
ICING:
225 g (8 oz/1½ cups) icing sugar
3-4 teaspoons water
few drops food colouring (optional)
tiny sweets, sugar strands, glacé cherries, or other cake
   decorations, to finish

Preheat oven to 180C (350F/Gas 4). In a bowl, mix together all the cake ingredients.

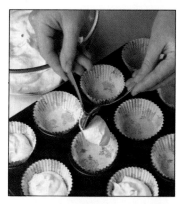

Using a teaspoon, divide the mixture between 20 paper bun cases placed in a tartlet tin. Bake in the oven for 15 minutes until golden. Transfer the cakes to a wire rack to cool before icing them.

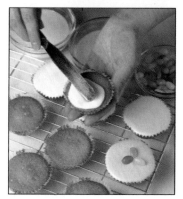

To make the icing, sift the icing sugar into a bowl and mix in enough water to give a smooth coating consistency. Tint some of the icing with a small amount of colouring, if liked. Spread the icing over the tops of the cakes and decorate as wished while the icing is still soft. Leave to set before serving.

Makes 20.

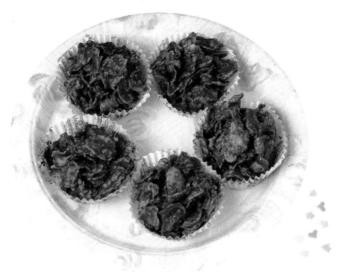

———————— CRISPY CRACKLES ————————

55 g (2 oz/¼ cup) margarine or butter
2 tablespoons golden syrup
115 g (4 oz) milk chocolate
85 g (3 oz/3 cups) cornflakes

Put the butter or margarine, syrup and chocolate into a medium saucepan and heat gently until the chocolate melts.

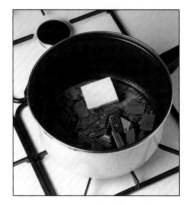

Remove the pan from the heat and stir in the cornflakes. Stir until the cornflakes are evenly coated.

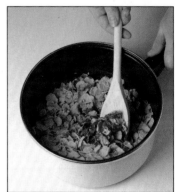

Put 12 paper bun cases into a tartlet tin and spoon in the cornflake mixture. Leave in the refrigerator until set.

Makes 12.

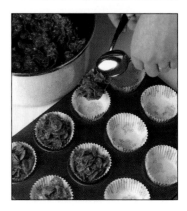

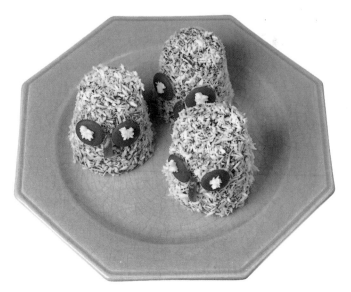

——OWL MADELEINES——

115 g (4 oz/½ cup) soft margarine
115 g (4 oz/½ cup) caster sugar
115 g (4 oz/1 cup) self-raising flour
2 eggs, beaten
few drops vanilla essence
4 tablespoons strawberry or raspberry jam
55 g (2 oz/⅔ cup) desiccated coconut
25 g (1 oz/6 teaspoons) butter
55 g (2 oz/⅓ cup) icing sugar
16 chocolate buttons
2 glacé cherries

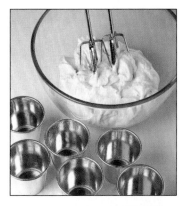

Grease 8 dariole moulds. Put margarine, sugar, flour, eggs and essence into a bowl and mix until smooth.

Preheat oven to 180C (350F/Gas 4). Spoon the cake mixture into the moulds, to come halfway up each one. Place on a baking sheet and bake in the oven for 15-18 minutes until cakes feel firm on top. Remove from the oven, run a knife round the sides of the moulds and turn onto a wire rack to cool. Trim the wider bases so the madeleines are all the same height.

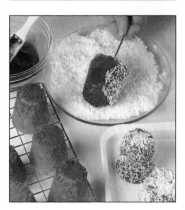

Melt the jam with 1 tablespoon water. Push a skewer into each cake, brush with jam then roll in the coconut until well coated. Put the cakes, narrower ends up, on a plate. Beat the butter and icing sugar together and use a little to attach 2 chocolate buttons to each cake for 'eyes' and pipe a spot in the middle of each. Complete the 'owls' with a piece of cherry to resemble the beak.

Makes 8.

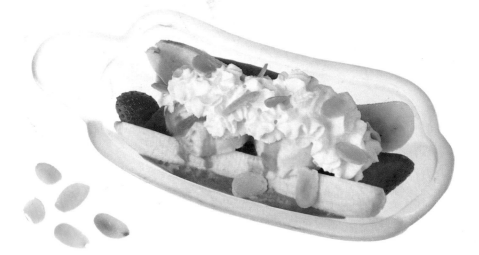

BANANA SPLITS

55 g (2 oz) fudge-filled chocolate bars
6 tablespoons single (light) cream
4 ripe bananas
a little lemon juice
8 large strawberries, sliced
8 scoops ice cream (vanilla or toffee fudge) flavour
whipped cream in aerosol can
1 tablespoon flaked almonds, lightly toasted

For the sauce, break the fudge-filled choco-late bars into small pieces and put into a small bowl with the single (light) cream. Place over a pan of simmering water and stir until completely melted and smooth.

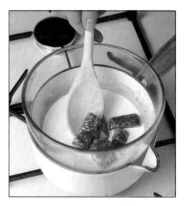

Cut the bananas in half lengthways and brush with a little lemon juice. Arrange in 4 long serving dishes and place a layer of straw-berries down the centre. Place 2 scoops of ice cream in each dish.

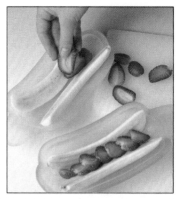

Drizzle over the fudge sauce, add a little aero-sol cream and finish with a scattering of flaked almonds.

Serves 4.

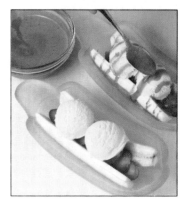

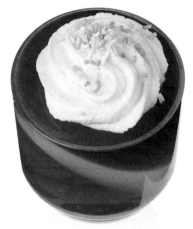

HARLEQUIN JELLIES

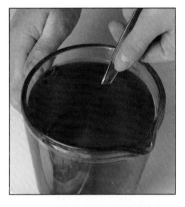

one 150 g (5 oz) red jelly (strawberry or raspberry
   flavour)
one 150 g (5 oz) yellow jelly (lemon or pineapple
   flavour)
one 150 g (5 oz) purple jelly (blackcurrant or black
   cherry flavour)
150 ml (5 fl oz/⅔ cup) whipping cream
sugar strands, or hundreds and thousands, to decorate

Make up the 3 jellies according to the direc-
tions on the packet.

Pour the red jelly into 6 tall plastic glasses
about 250 ml (9 fl oz/1 cup) capacity. (Plastic
picnic wine glasses are ideal.) Place them in
the refrigerator in a plastic box so that they
are tilted, a piece of kitchen roll placed on
the edge will stop them slipping. Leave
until set.

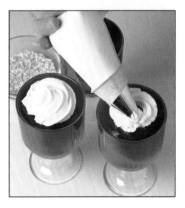

Pour the yellow jelly over the set red jelly,
and carefully prop the glasses a little more
upright, but still on a tilt. Leave until set.
Stand the jellies upright and pour in the
remaining purple jelly. Return to the refrigerator to set. Before serving, whip the cream,
pipe it on top of the jellies and scatter over
the sugar decoration.

Makes 6.

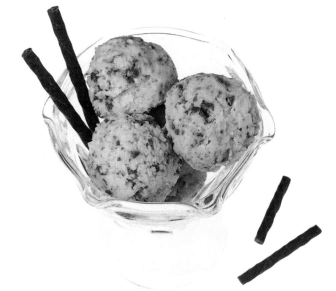

— MINT CHOC CHIP ICE CREAM —

1 tablespoon custard powder
2 tablespoons caster sugar
300 ml (10 fl oz/1¼ cups) milk
175 g (6 oz) can evaporated milk, chilled
few drops peppermint essence
few drops green food colouring
85 g (3 oz) plain (dark) chocolate, either chopped or
   grated
chocolate sticks, to serve (optional)

Blend custard powder and sugar with 2 table-spoons of the milk in a small saucepan. Stir in remaining milk and cook over a low heat until the custard thickens. Remove from the heat and pour into a bowl.

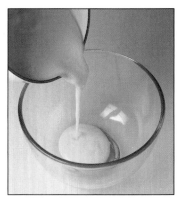

Cover the surface with a piece of greaseproof paper or cling film to prevent a skin from forming. Allow to cool. Whisk the evaporated milk until very thick, add the peppermint essence and food colouring. Fold into the custard then pour into a shallow container and place in freezer.

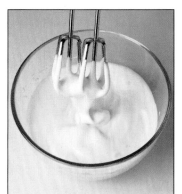

When the ice cream is set about 2.5 cm (1 in) all around the edge, turn into a bowl and whisk until smooth. Fold in the chocolate then return to a container and freeze until firm. To serve, transfer the ice cream to the refrigerator for 30 minutes to soften before scooping into bowls or glasses. Serve with chocolate sticks, if wished.

Serves 4-6.

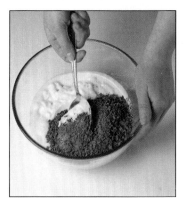

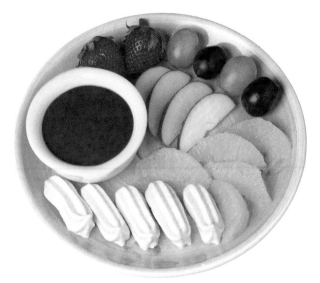

—MILK CHOCOLATE FONDUE—

225 g (8 oz) milk chocolate
150 ml (5 fl oz/²⁄₃ cup) single (light) cream
4 tablespoons orange juice
MERINGUES:
2 egg whites
115 g (4 oz/¹⁄₂ cup) caster sugar
a selection of fresh fruit, to serve

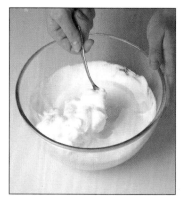

First, make the meringues. Preheat oven to 110C (225F/Gas ¼). Line 2 baking sheets with non-stick paper. Whisk the egg whites until stiff, then fold in half the sugar and whisk again until stiff. Lightly fold in the remaining sugar.

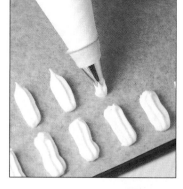

Put the meringue into a piping bag fitted with a small star nozzle and pipe small fingers onto the lined baking sheets. Bake in the oven for 1½-2 hours until they are crisp. Turn off the oven but leave the meringues in the oven to cool. Peel the meringues off the paper once they are cool.

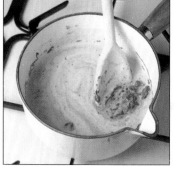

To make the fondue, break the chocolate into pieces and place in a saucepan. Add the cream and orange juice and heat gently until melted, stirring all the time. Pour into a warm serving dish and serve with the meringue fingers and fruit.

Serves 6-8.

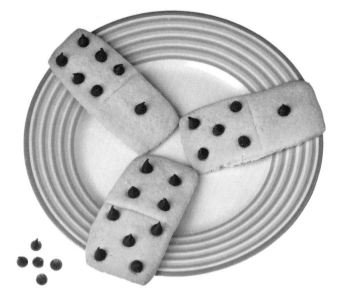

——————— DOMINO BISCUITS ———————

225 g (8 oz/2 cups) self-raising flour
115 g (4 oz/½ cup) butter or block margarine
115 g (4 oz/½ cup) caster sugar
finely grated rind 1 lemon
1 small egg, beaten
115 g (4 oz) packet plain (dark) chocolate drops

Preheat oven to 180C (350F/Gas 4). Sift the
flour into a bowl and rub in the butter until
the mixture resembles breadcrumbs. Stir in
the sugar and lemon rind, then mix to form a
dough with the egg. Turn onto a floured
surface and knead until smooth.

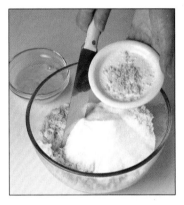

Roll the dough out to a rectangle about 0.5
cm (¼ in) thick. Cut into bars about 7.5 ×
4 cm (3 × 1½ in) and transfer to greased
baking sheets.

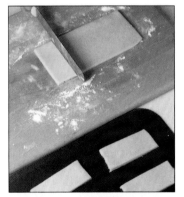

Mark each bar in half with a knife and
arrange chocolate drops on each one to
resemble domino dots. Bake in the oven for
12-15 minutes. Cool slightly before transfer-
ring to a wire rack to cool completely.

Makes about 20.

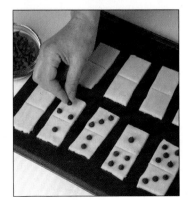

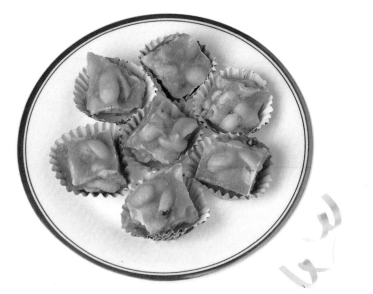

PEANUT BRITTLE

175 g (6 oz) skinned, unsalted peanuts
350 g (12 oz) granulated sugar
3 tablespoons golden syrup
25 g (1 oz/6 teaspoons) butter
pinch bicarbonate of soda

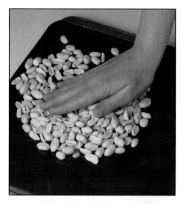

Lightly oil a 17.5 cm (7 in) shallow square tin. Spread the peanuts on a baking sheet and warm in the oven at 140C (275F/Gas 1) for about 15 minutes.

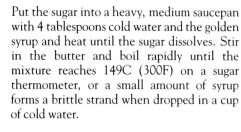

Put the sugar into a heavy, medium saucepan with 4 tablespoons cold water and the golden syrup and heat until the sugar dissolves. Stir in the butter and boil rapidly until the mixture reaches 149C (300F) on a sugar thermometer, or a small amount of syrup forms a brittle strand when dropped in a cup of cold water.

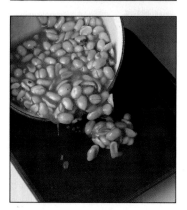

Remove from the heat, stir in the bicarbonate of soda and the peanuts. Pour into the tin and leave to cool. When almost set, mark into squares with an oiled knife. Break into pieces once set and wrap them in coloured cellophane, if wished.

Makes about 25 pieces.

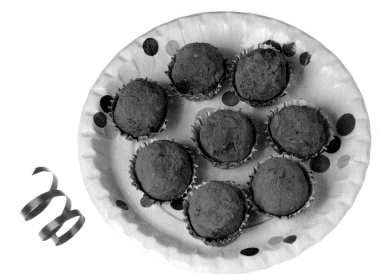

CHOCOLATE BALLS

115 g (4 oz/½ cup) butter
3 tablespoons golden syrup
115 g (4 oz) plain (dark) chocolate
85 g (3 oz) ready-to-eat apricots, chopped
175 g (6 oz) muesli-style cereal
drinking chocolate powder

Put the butter and golden syrup into a saucepan and heat gently until melted.

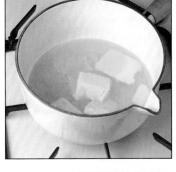

Break the chocolate into pieces, add to the pan and leave to melt. Beat together until smooth, then add the apricots and muesli; mix well. When cool, chill in the refrigerator for about 1 hour.

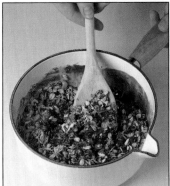

Take teaspoons of the mixture and roll into balls. Toss in the drinking chocolate, then place in petits fours cases. Return to the refrigerator until firm.

Makes about 20.

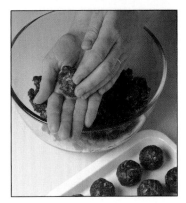

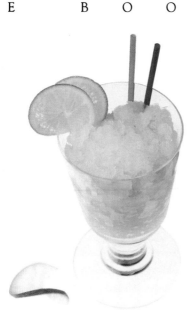

——— TROPICAL FRUIT CRUSH ———

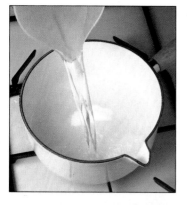

85 g (3 oz/⅓ cup) sugar
2 passion fruit
1 ripe mango, peeled and chopped
juice 1 orange
slices orange or lime, to serve

Put the sugar into a saucepan with 450 ml
(16 fl oz/2 cups) water. Bring to the boil and
simmer for 5 minutes. Set aside to cool.

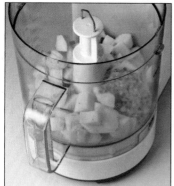

Scoop out the flesh from the passion fruit and
put into a blender or food processor with the
mango and orange juice and blend to a purée,
then sieve. Stir in the cooled sugar syrup,
pour into a shallow tray and place the mixture
in the freezer.

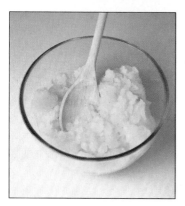

Stir the mixture at regular intervals during
freezing and continue to freeze until it has the
texture of coarse crystals without being frozen
solid. Empty into a chilled bowl and crush the
mixture to break it down to small crystals.
Return to the tray and freeze again until ready
to serve. Spoon into glasses and decorate
with orange or lime slices.

Serves about 6.

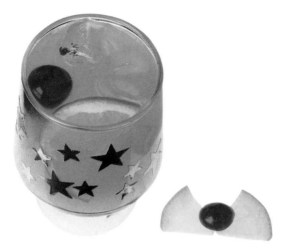

── SPARKLING FRUIT PUNCH ──

2 oranges
200 g (7 oz) can pineapple pieces in juice
2 tablespoons maraschino cherries
1 litre (35 fl oz/4½ cups) orange juice
450 ml (16 fl oz/2 cups) pineapple juice
1 litre (35 fl oz/4½ cups) lemonade
ice cubes

Slice the oranges, cut in half and put into a large bowl with the pineapple, its juice and the cherries.

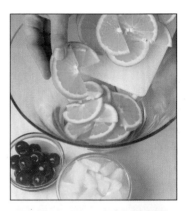

Pour over the orange juice and pineapple juice and leave in the refrigerator until ready to serve.

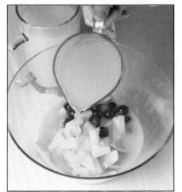

Just before serving, add the lemonade and ice cubes; stir. Serve in glasses and make sure a little fruit is added to each.

Serves about 10.

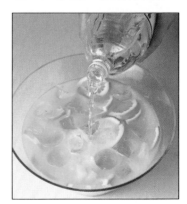

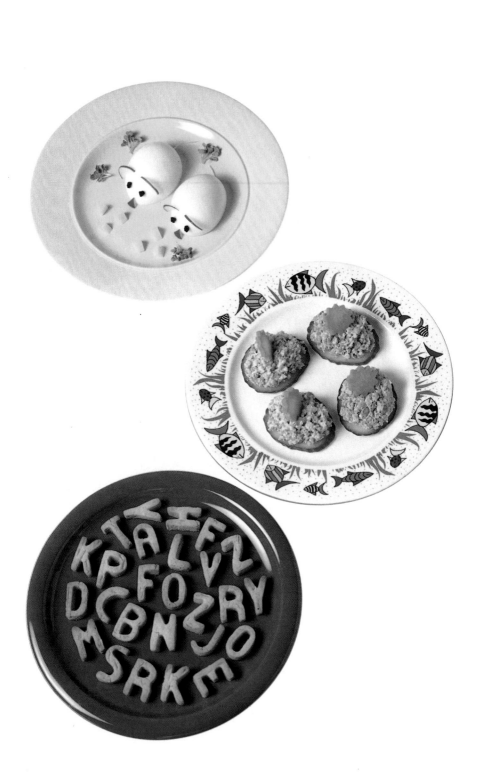

CHEESY MICE
page 29

CUCUMBER SNACKS
page 54

ALPHABET BISCUITS
page 27

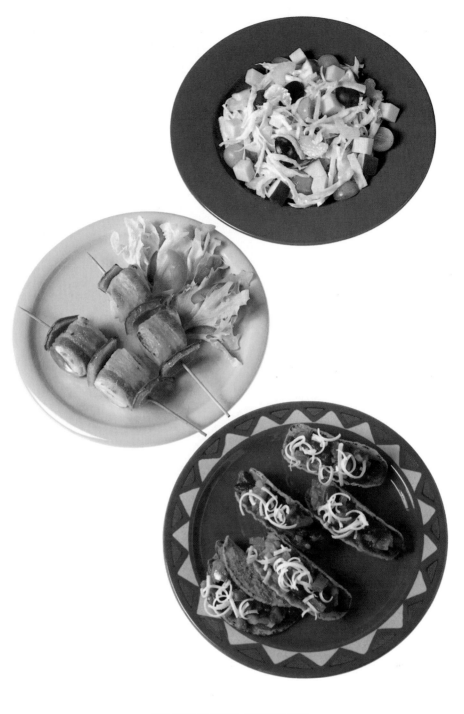

FRUITY CHEESE COLESLAW
page 43

BANANA & BACON ROLLS
page 41

MINI TACOS
page 39

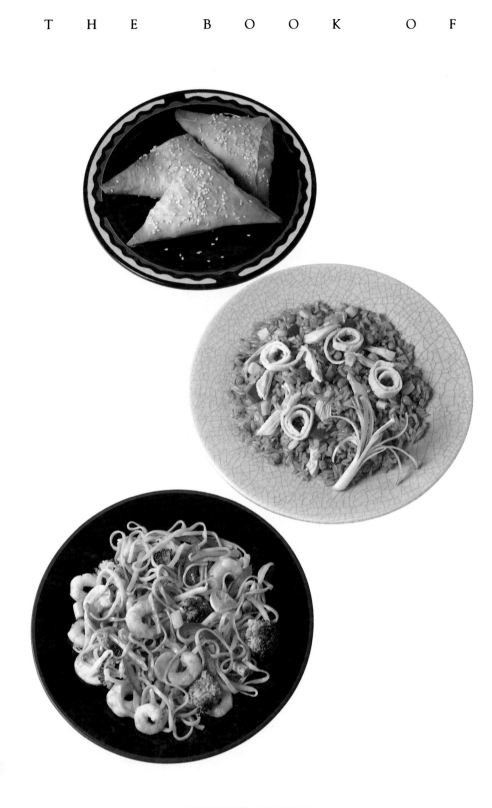

VEGETABLE SAMOSAS
page 74

CHICKEN FRIED RICE
page 81

CHOP SUEY SALAD
page 63

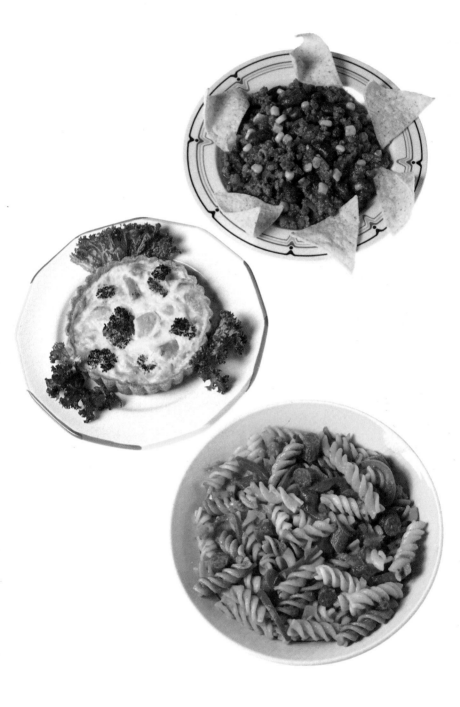

MEXICAN SUPPER
page 75

TURKEY & BROCCOLI FLANS
page 72

PEPPERAMI PASTA
page 66

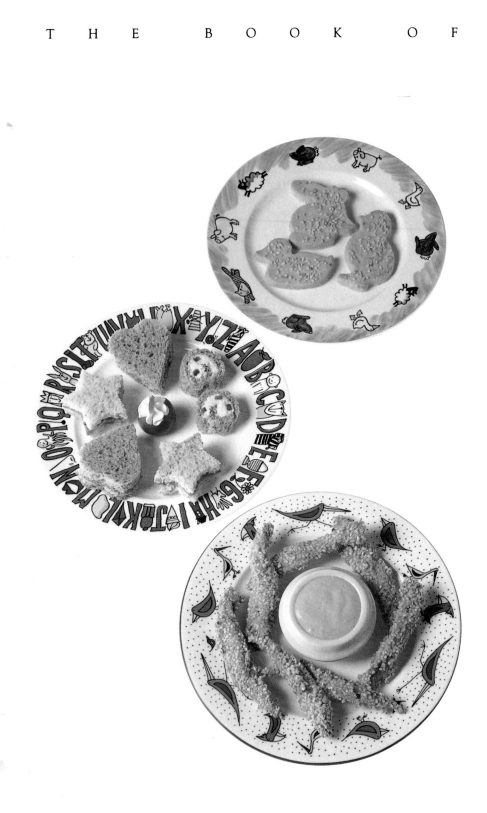

ANIMAL CHEESE BISCUITS
page 91

PARTY SANDWICHES
page 87

SESAME CHICKEN FINGERS
page 92